Surviving

Cancer

SURPRISED BY LIFE!

by Carol Nylander

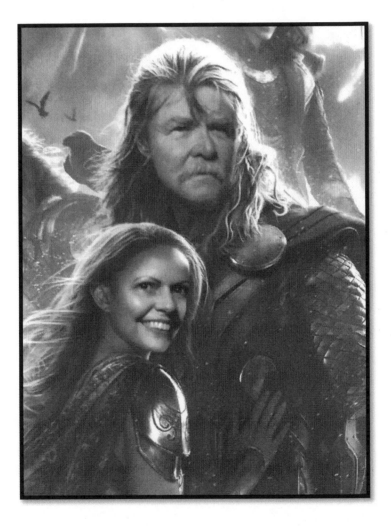

Comical post-cancer photo of Morris and I
just for the fun of it; celebrating life!

INTRODUCTION

I have no real interest in the topic of cancer, and I'm certain most people would prefer to avoid it entirely. It's an unpleasant subject, and reviewing my experiences with cancer has been difficult. There are so many more enjoyable and interesting things to talk about.

But for someone who against their will has been abruptly plunged into the bewildering world of cancer, the subject suddenly takes on urgent importance, because it must. Life and death decisions must be made with little time to deliberate. As we were initially trying to make treatment decisions we were presented with multiple treatment options, and some were in direct opposition to each other. Obviously we could not try them all.

As a cancer survivor I know exactly how baffling and overwhelming that feels. I myself began that glum journey on March 21st, 2014 with a diagnosis of stage IV ovarian cancer. Instantaneously my normal life was turned upside down, and everything revolved around only one thing; cancer. Cancer was not a subject I wanted to know about, but it was essential to learn, and fast.

It is my hope that if cancer has become an unpleasant reality for you or someone you love, you will find help and encouragement in this book from someone who has walked through the gloom, and back into the light. At one point my health had declined to the point that no one, including myself thought I could possibly recover, and yet, I was "Surprised by life."

I am a Christian, and my faith in God played an indispensable role in my recovery. I want to share how and why my faith in Christ comforted and supported me; and why it would have done so whether I recovered or not.

Because we no longer live in a world where Christianity is the dominant world view I cannot assume that everyone will understand what I mean when I use terms like 'faith' or 'God.' When I use the words 'faith' and 'God,' I am speaking of my unshakable confidence and trust (faith) in the Supreme Being, the creator and ruler of everything as described in the Bible. The Bible teaches that there is only one God, but He is exists as three in one, Father, Son (Jesus Christ) and Holy Spirit. When I say 'God' that is specifically who I am referring to.

This account of my battle with cancer is uniquely mine, so I am the person best qualified to tell it. But the comfort I received from faith in Jesus Christ during a period of deep distress has been shared by countless millions in innumerable difficult situations. Though many others are better qualified to explain it than I, in this book I have tried to communicate it for the benefit of others. My big 'take away' from the cancer ordeal is that you never know how important your faith in God is, until that is about all you have left.

"Praise be to the God and Father of our Lord Jesus Christ, the Father of compassion and the God of all comfort, who comforts us in all our troubles, *so that we can comfort those in any trouble with the comfort we ourselves receive from God.*" [1]

[1] 2 CORINTHIANS 1:3-4 (NLT). MOST BIBLE REFERENCES ARE TAKEN FROM THE NEW LIVING TRANSLATION (NLT)

I received comfort from God and in this book I hope to share that comfort with others who are also struggling with cancer, or any other problem beyond their control.

ACKNOWLEGEMENTS

I doubt I would still be here today without the prayers, tangible assistance and moral support of numerous people.

My friend, Sandy Stein, repeatedly encouraged me to tell the story of my fight with cancer, and this book would probably not exist without her urging.

I would especially like to thank my husband, best friend, and caretaker, Morris, who labored tirelessly to help me every step of the way. He also edited this book and his comments and observations resulted in a vast improvement to my original writings.

✱ Cover photos are actual photos of me (Carol) first taken during my cancer struggle and again after my recovery. I used the Pic Collage app to modify them to resemble black and white drawings but I think the original, unmodified photo makes me look even worse than the one on the cover if you can believe that. Cancer nearly killed me, and a picture is worth a 1,000 words!

SPECIAL THANKS

My doctors; Dr. Cervantes, Dr. Stewart, Dr. Rajendra, Dr. Steves, Dr. Belote and Dr. Tuan Nguyen for their excellent care.

For all the prayers, meals and support provided by members of Purcellville Baptist Church, and Cornerstone Chapel in Leesburg.

My coworkers at the Town of Leesburg who shared their leave with me, brought meals, visited me, and encouraged me in many other ways.

All my friends and family who helped in very tangible ways, starting with my cousins; Ken & Tim Schilke, Terrie Schilke May, Inger Ueland, and friends; Ellen Sprague, Bill Lolli, Anne Bittner, Paul & Barbara Farner and their daughter, Jolene Knudsen, Arthur Estes, Paula & Mike White, Dave Charlton, John Shaw, and many others, too numerous to mention.

Thanks to countless others who helped in big ways or small. Some people told me they prayed for me every night; others who didn't even know me brought a meal. Some visited me in the hospital. Others sent cards or flowers. Experiencing the generous kindness of both friends and strangers was one of the truly good things about having a life threatening illness.

My sincere love and gratitude to them all!

TABLE OF CONTENTS

CHAPTER 1

THE LONG, DARK ROAD

"I'm sorry to have to tell you this, but you have stage IV ovarian cancer," said the nurse. That's how I first learned that I was in for the fight of my life. It would be a fight for life itself, and a journey I certainly did not want to take. It was Friday evening, March 21, 2014, my own personal 'date that will live in infamy.' In the previous months I had become increasingly lethargic, which was very unlike me. I've always been an extremely healthy person, rarely even getting a cold. Feeling good has always been normal to me. So at the age of 60 when I found myself huffing and puffing when climbing the stairs at work, I attributed it to getting older.

But at this point I was way beyond tired. I was completely drained of all energy. The previous two weekends found me sleeping 2 days and 3 nights straight and I could have easily continued sleeping for the foreseeable future. I couldn't understand it. That had never happened before! I wondered if I had the flu but there were no symptoms other than total exhaustion.

By this time we had been living in Virginia for 10 years and I still didn't even have a family doctor! I was always healthy, so it felt like a waste of time and money. I did take care of my health, just not by going to the doctors. That probably sounds negligent and I don't recommend following my bad example, but that was the way I functioned. I have avoided doctors as much as possible all my life. But that was about to change, and soon my life would revolve around doctor appointments and unfamiliar medical tests and procedures. I would become acquainted with medical terms I wish I never needed to know.

Nevertheless, I've been told by doctors that even if I had been having regular checkups it would be very unlikely that my ovarian cancer would have been detected any earlier. It's often mistaken for an upset stomach or bowel problems and it is very common that it is not revealed for what it is until the cancer is in an advanced stage. Unfortunately there are not a lot of reliable screening tests for ovarian cancer.

Medical information doesn't interest me much, but I am very thankful that lots of other good people have studied Medicine and learned ways to help others. By now I have more than made up for my former lack of doctor visits with all the numerous doctor appointments I've had since being diagnosed. I still don't enjoy going to the doctor, but now I realize the necessity of it.

As another weekend approached, I could tell I would again be sleeping continuously. I was so tired that I had even been napping in the car during my lunch break. Even though I tended to avoid doctors it became apparent to even me that I needed to see a doctor. The doctor we selected (Dr. Belote) said he couldn't get me in until Monday. He recommended that I go over to Cornwall Hospital in Leesburg after work to get a CAT scan because he said he would want to have a CAT scan to look at when he saw me anyway.

So my husband, Morris, met me at the hospital after work and I started drinking barium which helps to show up parts of the body not always clearly visible on scans, like blood vessels, the kidneys and liver. Barium is flavored but chalky and not easy to get down. It needs time to take effect so I slowly drank, and we waited.

Later in the evening they finally got around to taking the scan and then sent the results to Washington, D.C. to be read. We waited some more. We had arrived around 5:30 PM and Morris had been with me the entire time. Around 10:00 PM he needed to use the restroom and almost as soon as he left, the nurse came in with the results of the scan. We had been waiting together for 5 hours, and now that I was alone in the room for the first time all night, the nurse walked in, which was an odd coincidence! She said, "We received the results of your CAT scan. I'm sorry to have to tell you this, but you have stage IV ovarian cancer."

In retrospect, one of the most interesting things about that experience was my reaction. I wasn't scared, moved to tears or even upset. My dominant thought was, "How bizarre!" I was the healthiest person I knew; never got sick, didn't smoke or drink and tried hard to eat healthy food and exercise. I was a few pounds over my ideal weight but other than that I didn't do anything bad for my health, and did do everything possible to promote good health. So it seemed inconceivable that I should have stage IV cancer. It felt surreal, unreal, like being in the Twilight Zone, or like just being told that my face is blue. But there it was; stage IV ovarian cancer.

Just about when the nurse and I had finished talking, Morris returned to the room and I asked her if she could repeat what she told me so he could hear it. So I heard it again; Stage IV ovarian cancer. Unbelievable! It was baffling, perplexing, mystifying, but what struck me later was the complete absence of fear.

The nurse said they would arrange an appointment for me with an oncologist and we could go home. Morris and I were a little bewildered. Information of this magnitude is hard to assimilate and we had not had time to process it. So we passively accepted the appointment with the unknown doctor and went home.

ANNE

We prayed about it and the next day, Saturday, we began to gather as much information as we could in order to make the best decisions possible. We thought about people we knew who had dealt with cancer, wanting to learn what they thought had been helpful and what they would have done differently. We hoped that a common thread would emerge yielding clues for the best approach to attack cancer.

We began by calling Anne who lived very nearby. Anne's husband, Tim, had battled cancer for a little less than three years. They discovered his cancer in March 2011 and he passed away in January 2014, just a couple of months before we found out I had cancer. Though Anne was still grieving from her recent loss she kindly welcomed us to come over and talk to her for a couple of hours.

Anne and Tim had taken a combination approach to combating cancer. In addition to following the oncologist's recommendations exactly, they added nutritional supplements, juicing and anything that might strengthen Tim's body for the fight.

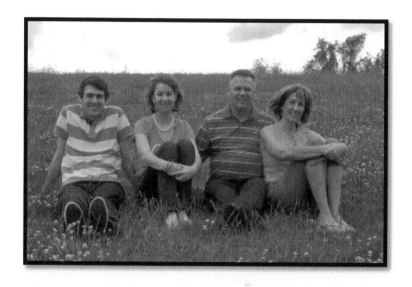

Tim and his family in healthier times;
Nathan, Ashley, Tim & Anne

Tim was a remarkable human being. In the fall of 2012 while he was in an advanced stage of cancer, he was still volunteering as a lay pastor with Samaritan's Purse. He was ministering to others in New Jersey and New York who had recently lost their homes and property due to Hurricane Sandy. Morris and I were visiting with him just before he was about to leave for that mission trip and he expressed how glad he was that he had recently had his ascites drained so that he would be better able to serve others! I now know what ascites feels like, and I am amazed that he had the strength, ability or even the inclination to do it.

The first time I ever heard the word "ascites" was from Tim. We all have a certain amount of fluid cycling through our abdomens, enough to keep the organs lubricated. But the fluids don't get trapped there, they move along. By contrast, ascites are fluids that accumulate inside the abdomen. They cannot escape and the abdomen continues to expand to make room for it, creating a lot of pressure and discomfort.

I had a desk job so prior to getting sick I tried to squeeze in a little exercise at every opportunity. I walked up the stairs instead of taking the elevator. I didn't look for the closest parking space because I didn't mind walking a few extra steps, and I usually did about 100 sit-ups at night. I had stopped doing sit-ups about a month before I was diagnosed because my abdomen felt odd (not painful, just abnormal and a little uncomfortable). The best I can describe it is that it felt like a lot of fluid was sloshing around in my abdomen. As I later learned, that's exactly what it was. I didn't know it at that time but I had ascites. Tim had explained to me what ascites were, and now I had them too! At the time I was diagnosed, March 21, 2014, I was already at stage IV with ascites.

Ascites causes a great deal of pressure and discomfort. The only way to get relief is to have the fluid drained at a hospital in a process called paracentesis. A doctor makes a perforation in the abdomen with a hollow needle to drain the fluid, which can amount to many liters. It's not extremely painful, but it is uncomfortable.

Ascites can be caused by a variety of things but it is a symptom found in advanced stages of some cancers. These fluids aren't just water, they also contain proteins and much needed nutrients. So when they are drained away, they are also draining away much needed nourishment.

Just months before Tim died he was volunteering again with Samaritan's Purse in Lyons, Colorado after a major flood in that area. He led three people to the Lord on that trip. Incredibly, even while his own life was slipping away, he was still serving others!

Tim had to have his ascites drained fairly often. Eventually it got to the point that there were multiple pockets of ascites in his abdomen and they could no longer drain them all. Sadly, he passed away shortly after his 55th birthday, leaving behind his wife, Anne, and their two teenaged children, Nathan and Ashley.

RITA

The next day, Sunday, we called Rita. We really did not know Rita very well at that point in time, but though we were relative strangers she was extremely supportive! She was the next door neighbor of our good friend, Eddie, and that's how we learned about her struggle with cervical cancer. When first diagnosed she had done exactly what her gynecologist told her to do which included a very intrusive use of radioactive rods. After the first unpleasant treatment, she reconsidered. The treatment sounded extreme and pretty crazy to her.

Instead she made an appointment with a naturopathic doctor, and went in an entirely different direction. A naturopathic doctor relies on natural methods rather than traditional Western Medicine. Rita's gynecologist scolded, threatened, intimidated and tried every tactic to get Rita to return for more radiation treatments but Rita steadfastly refused.

By the time we talked with her, Rita was doing extremely well. She was eating organic food and receiving a variety of alternative cancer therapies, mostly treatments that were not covered by insurance. It was very costly, but Rita felt better about the approach she was taking, and her only regret was that she had one conventional treatment with the radioactive rods. She was concerned about the damage that exposure to radiation may have already done. Rita was so kind, and she sat with us on her front porch on that pleasant day in early spring, answering all our questions until we couldn't think of anything else to ask her. At that time Rita was in radiant health and it was obvious that her natural approach was effective. She was in remission.

Rita only lived a couple of miles from our house but when I was hospitalized at Medstar Hospital in Washington, D.C., she drove all the way there to visit me! She could have waited and conveniently visited me just about any other time, because she lived so nearby. I guess Washington, D.C. isn't the end of the earth, but it is a long drive and I was astonished that she came that far to see me.

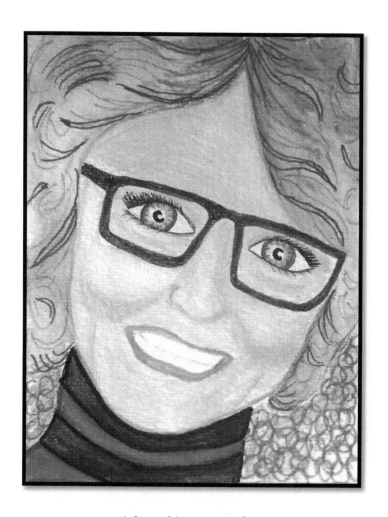

I drew this portrait of Rita,
for her memorial gathering in
April, 2018

Much later after I recovered from cancer we saw Rita periodically at our small Post Office in Round Hill and she always looked terrific. The last time we saw her at the Post Office was toward the end of 2017, glowing as usual with her big, friendly grin.

So I was horrified when six weeks later at the beginning of 2018, Rita called to ask me how to manage ascites. I couldn't believe she was experiencing ascites. It is a late stage symptom of cancer! I came over as quickly as I could only to find that she was already receiving hospice care in her living room! It made my head spin to see how quickly her vibrant health deteriorated to being on hospice care. It seemed unreal, like a nightmare.

Her health quickly declined, and she soon realized it was futile to fight it. I tried to persuade her to keep trying, but after hearing her perspective, I realized that she was just too debilitated. She wanted to continue to fight; she just had no more strength. Sadly, the day after I last spoke with her, Rita passed away.

We met Rita in 2012 and she passed away at the beginning of 2018. During all the time we knew her she was always cheerful, willing to help in any way possible and vibrantly healthy. How could this have happened? I asked Rita that question and her only response was that she had been under a lot of stress; not from her family, her relationships were healthy, so I don't really know what caused the stress. But that is the only thing she could point to that could have caused her cancer to revive and overpower her.

It doesn't seem like stress would be enough to kill a person, but apparently it is. I guess the mind and body are so busy coping with stress that they are diverted from exclusively fighting cancer. Whatever the cause, my beautiful, kind friend was gone.

So the question remains, was it a good idea to use alternative treatments, such as high dose Vitamin C, along with juicing and organic eating? Or would Rita have been better off to go with conventional medicine? That question can never be answered with certainty, at least not to my satisfaction.

Every type of cancer is different and requires different treatment. Every person is different and how their body responds to the treatments will not be exactly the same in every case. My oncologist later told me that I was in the top .01% of responders to the chemo he selected for me. That's really great, but it also means that 99.9% of his patients don't have that kind of excellent response. One size does not fit all when it comes to cancer. For that reason it's difficult to make a decision on how to best treat it. It's such an important life and death decision, and as laypeople Morris and I were really not equipped to evaluate our options with much confidence. We did not have a lot of time to make our decision either!

Rita chose alternative medicine, relying on naturopathic (natural) treatments and for several years it appeared obvious that it was the right decision, until inexplicably her health completely collapsed in a few short weeks.

DR. BELOTE

On Monday our first doctor visit was with my new General Practitioner, Dr. Belote. Doctors are under a lot of pressure to treat patients in a brief window of time so sometimes it's hard to get all your questions answered unless they were well thought out in advance. But when we told Dr. Belote of my diagnosis it was as if I was his only patient that day and he patiently answered every question we could think of until we ran out of things to ask.

I can't remember exactly how long we were in his office, but I suspect it was an hour or more. Before we left he asked if it would be alright if he prayed for us and of course we said 'yes!' We had found the perfect doctor, for us anyway. When we returned to the waiting room it was crowded with patients because our appointment with Dr. Belote lasted so much longer than what would normally be expected.

From very early on I observed that unfailingly people generously gave of their time, immediately and for as long as we desired their attention. I suppose it was because my diagnosis was so life-threatening that they realized that whatever I needed had to be dealt with immediately. They always seemed to understand that getting back to me in a few weeks might truly be too late. It is amazing how kind and helpful people can be, even relative strangers, and experiencing their consistent kindness was a comfort.

Dr. Belote's primary recommendation was to 'eat well'. Morris and I perked up at that recommendation because we thought his suggestion meant that eating really well (juicing, organic food, etc.) was somehow a treatment in itself, but that was not what he meant at all. When we asked for specific guidelines, he had none to offer, except to 'eat well.' That was a bit puzzling at the time but much farther along in my cancer journey I understood why he advised me to 'eat well'.

We later learned from my oncologist that cancer depends on its host for sustenance and takes what it wants first and the patient gets whatever is left which turns out to be very little. Because of that my weight continued to plummet. Normally I would have been glad to lose weight, but this was uncontrollable weight loss. If I had died from cancer, most likely the actual cause of death would have been starvation, but cancer would be the reason why I was starving. That is why Dr. Belote advised me to 'eat well.'

Just today (as I write this) we saw Dr. Belote, probably for the last time because he is retiring. In our parting visit he told us that he is really a very shy, introverted person and his vocation as a doctor allowed him to meet and interact with many more people than he would have otherwise. He also mentioned that as a Christian, he strove to use his calling as a Christian ministry, blessing and serving others. He truly did bless and serve me and I'm glad that I am still around to be able to thank him for his excellent care and the time he lavished on a new patient in the most serious health crisis of her life.

DR. AMY

At Cornwall Hospital on the night I received the news that I had cancer, the nurse made an appointment for me with some random, unknown oncologist, and we said, okay. So we had no previous knowledge of Dr. Amy; we didn't choose her, in fact we had never heard of her before that night. She was nice enough; in fact there was a plaque on the wall of her office that said that she had been voted 'the kindest doctor' the previous year. I thought that was a good sign, it couldn't hurt anyway. However we didn't really feel a rapport with her, but we tried to listen with an open mind.

I told her that I would like to know the whole truth, even if it was hard to hear. So she gave me an honest assessment of how serious my diagnosis was. She probably was more direct than she would normally be, and told us more than most doctors would have. However, that was what I asked for and we appreciated her frankness. She said that by definition Stage IV Ovarian cancer is incurable, so the goal would only be to prolong my life. If I did nothing, she predicted I might not be around by Christmas. But if I followed the chemo, surgery, then more chemo regimen, I would have an 18% chance of being around in 5 years. That did not seem like much of a success story to me. An 18% chance seems pretty small, less than 1 out of 5 chances for survival!

For quite some time prior to having cancer we had felt suspicious of mainstream medicine's strict reliance upon cutting, burning and poisoning (surgery, radiation, chemo) and we had grown uncomfortable with that approach. Plus there is such a phenomenal amount of money being made on pharmaceuticals. With that much money in play, we doubted that physicians' lavish use of pharmaceuticals was completely necessary or even beneficial.

We had been researching alternative therapies and in many ways the various natural therapies paralleled each other. A great deal of emphasis was placed on diet; no meat, dairy, sugar or any other foods that create an acidic environment favorable to cancer. Instead they emphasized fresh

22

vegetable juices and foods that create an alkaline environment which was hostile to cancer.

Exercise was encouraged because it increased oxygen, which cancer hates, along with lots of other complementary therapies that are safe and harmless; designed to fortify the immune system. That approach just made more sense to Morris and me. We knew this was a serious situation and that the cancer had to be attacked aggressively. But we felt much better about creating a hostile environment for cancer and strengthening the immune system than we did about poisonous chemicals that attack both the cancer and the body. That was our point of view at the beginning of all of this, and remained so for a long time to come.

Dr. Amy recommended six months of chemo treatments, then surgery, and more chemo. On April 1, 2014, eleven days after being diagnosed, Morris and I returned to Dr. Amy's office for a group orientation class to prepare us for chemo. It was surreal. About 10 people sat around a table with a big bowl of candy in the center (keep in mind, sugar feeds cancer) and we got a one hour briefing on what to expect from chemo therapy. The obvious assumption was that everyone there was planning to accept chemo treatments.

Dr. Amy's offices were on the second floor and had large picture windows with a pretty park-like view of trees and well-manicured lawns. Lined up facing out the windows were a long row of comfortable, spa type lounge chairs so the patients could gaze out the window at the attractive view as they were hooked up to a chemo drip. Chemo does kill cancer, but it also attacks other parts of the body, so it is a race to find out what will give out first, the cancer or the body. So to me it seemed creepy to sit in comfortable chairs looking at a beautiful view, while poison dripped into one's veins. Although Dr. Amy recommended chemo (which was what we had expected), at that time we were not comfortable with that option and decided not to do it.

FAMILY AND FRIENDS

Probably the most difficult thing about a new diagnosis of cancer is that you know you have to do something, and you know you have to do it fast. But you also realize that you don't know enough about cancer to identify where to start. Most people probably think that doing exactly what a doctor recommends is the best course, and I understand that reasoning. Doctors have years of education and experience, and that's why we seek their advice. But it's not their body they are working on, it's just a job, and they are not always right. We were not yet ready to blindly follow a doctor's advice. We were praying about it and doing our best to think this through.

Another aspect of having cancer was the difficult and painful necessity of informing family and friends of my diagnosis. To anyone who cared about me at all it would be hard news to hear. I would be the reason for their pain, whether I liked it or not, and I definitely did not like it. I called our son, Paul, but first I made sure he was not driving because I thought that could potentially be hazardous. He went home and told his wife, Catherine, and they both had a long cry.

My mother was 90 at the time, and her health had recently been declining in numerous ways. I did not want to accelerate her health problems by telling her about my illness. She tends to be rather emotional and I thought that news would be too much for her. There was nothing she could do to help, so I thought it would be best not to tell her. If I got better she would never need to know. I did in fact get better, and she still doesn't know about it.

I did not want to tell my sister, Lisa, over the phone while she might be home alone. I wanted her to have moral support. So I sent a letter from me to Lisa to be read in person by Lisa's friend, Debbie. I thought that it would be best if Lisa had the support of a trusted friend during such a difficult time. Nothing would really soften the blow, but I wanted to make it as easy on her as possible.

We also had to tell our daughter, Crystal. We told her while eating at a fast food restaurant. It was a calm conversation but I know she felt it deeply. It's just not the sort of news anyone wants to hear; not the patient, and not anyone who cares about them. Cancer is hard on everyone, not just the person who has it.

The majority of our relatives live in either California or Washington State. Our son, Paul and his wife, Catherine have young children. Even if anyone wished to help they still would not have been able to stay long and their help would be very limited. So we were going to be pretty much on our own, without help from family.

SHAWN

Thirdly we visited Shawn who was in remission from two unrelated cancers; meaning there was no cancer detectable. Originally she had been treated for colorectal cancer. After being successfully treated she had a PET scan. No colorectal cancer was detected, but now the scan revealed another completely unrelated cancer; Ovarian cancer! That is the same thing I had and it is called a 'silent killer' precisely because it doesn't present any symptoms until it is well advanced. That makes it extremely difficult to detect in an early stage. It is usually mistaken for stomach problems, bad digestion and similar issues that have nothing to do with cancer.

Usually it is discovered when it is already stage IV, which was when my cancer was discovered. Following that pattern Shawn did not have any symptoms and her ovarian cancer would have likely gone undetected until much later if she had not had a PET scan to check whether her colorectal cancer was gone. Some would call that a fortunate coincidence, but I consider it as God bringing good from a bad situation and so does Shawn.

Shawn is the wife of a pastor at Purcellville Baptist Church, and she was also generous with her time. Shawn and her husband, Pastor Kurt, took an entirely different approach. They did not do a lot of research when she was diagnosed, and stayed completely off the Internet. They felt that it would not be helpful and would only cause confusion. So they chose to let the Lord lead them and they relied entirely on her doctor's recommendations. She received conventional treatments, including chemotherapy, and she made a full recovery. I've seen Shawn recently and she is still in excellent health; cancer free for six years!

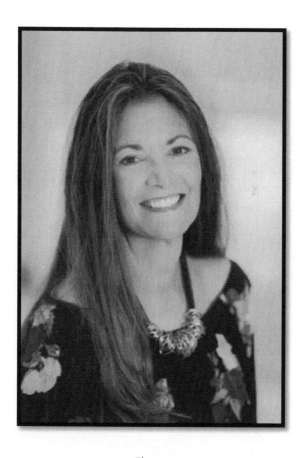

Shawn

When I had my second surgery in Washington, DC, Pastor Kurt and Shawn drove all the way there to pray with Morris and me before the operation. It's about 60 miles of congestion and traffic, so I marveled at every single visitor I received who was willing to make that trek.

Shawn chose conventional medicine and it appears that was the right choice, for her at least. That is the puzzling thing about making a decision regarding cancer treatments. Shawn chose conventional medicine and it worked. But since she didn't do all the things that Rita did there is no way to know if the treatments Rita received might also have worked for Shawn.

Conversely, Rita only received one conventional cancer treatment before abandoning it forever. Her naturopathic approach worked extremely well for several years and gave her an excellent quality of life, without any adverse side effects. But since she did not chose conventional medicine it can't be proven whether or not that would have been a better choice for her.

By now Morris and I had heard Rita's story of exclusively pursuing naturopathic treatments. After talking to her, that sounded pretty good. It appeared that it was probably the way to go. But then we talked to Shawn who exclusively pursued conventional medicine with excellent results, making that look like the best choice. We couldn't have it both ways; we had to choose one or the other.

In some ways talking to Rita and Shawn yielded a lot of helpful information, and in other ways it added to our confusion. We found that while researching, we came across many conflicting reports, such as, "you need to exercise daily to let your body know you want to live." And the next recommendation would be, "Your body needs to rest so it can heal." There is logic to both suggestions but it's impossible to do them both so selecting the best approach was a perplexing dilemma.

Rita used a natural approach which worked for a while until suddenly it didn't. Shawn used a conventional approach that was successful even to the present day. Tim used a combination approach which ultimately was not successful for him. Our visits to consult with friends had been both helpful and perplexing.

DR. STEWART

Next we spoke to Dr. Stewart, a medical doctor who preferred to rely as much as possible on natural treatments, as opposed to drugs and surgery. We were in his office for quite a long time, maybe two hours, talking and asking him questions. He informed us of treatments we could try. Most of them would require long drives, and none of them would be covered by insurance.

What we were finding was that if we opted for standard medical treatments, like chemo and surgery, they would be covered by insurance. If we wanted to try other, more natural and less intrusive options as Rita had done, we could not unless we paid for all of it out of pocket. Rita had good results for several years with the natural approach, but it was a huge financial drain. Rita felt the cost was worth it.

Dr. Stewart was helpful and knowledgeable, but also very expensive, and most of what he had to offer was not covered by insurance. If we opted to use Dr. Stewart as my primary doctor, it would cost a lot of money and we didn't have it.

Dr. Stewart made another important suggestion; that we should consult with an acupuncture doctor that he highly recommended, Dr. Tuan Anh Nguyen. Though he was highly recommended, at that point we did not go visit Dr. Nguyen's Acupuncture and Herb Clinic. I really wish we had! From this point on when referring to Dr. Nguyen I will refer to him by his first name, Dr. Tuan, because he is a very kind and amiable man, and I think of him more as a friend now. Later Dr. Tuan became one of my doctors and he was an enormous help. I will talk more about him later.

GERSON CLINIC

I had heard about the Gerson cancer treatment therapy long before I knew I had cancer, so we called them next. Dr. Max Gerson was a Jewish-German doctor who experienced terrible migraine headaches while in medical school. He asked the doctors and his fellow students how to treat migraines but nobody could help him. So in desperation he tried to come up with a way to treat himself by devising a special diet. He found that if he followed it carefully, the migraines were gone. Later he escaped Nazi Germany and immigrated to America. He discovered quite by accident that his special diet helped heal patients suffering from many other illnesses, including cancer, if the diet was strictly adhered to.

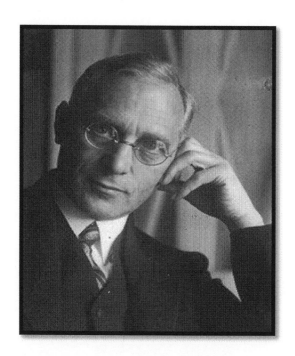

Dr. Max Gerson

However, he ran into a lot of opposition from the medical community and was not permitted to freely treat people with his method, even if they wanted it. Today the Gerson Therapy is still being used to treat cancer, but not in the United States. There is a Gerson Clinic in Tijuana, Mexico and people stay there for one, two or three weeks along with their caregiver to learn how to do everything necessary. It's a lot of work, it's not easy, and so a caregiver is required.

STEVE

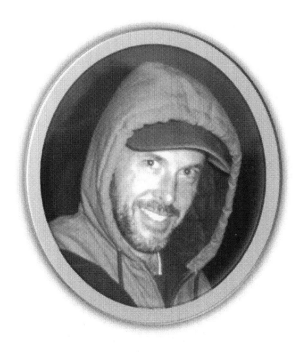

Four years earlier our views on cancer treatments significantly shifted toward naturopathic medicine after what happened to our good family friend, Steve, an outgoing, intelligent, and healthy young husband and father. He, his wife, Ellen and their two young children, Kyra and Aidan regularly attended the weekly Bible Study we had in our home. In January 2010 Steve began having hip pains and at first his doctor told him it was arthritis.

But the hip pain persisted and grew increasingly more intense. He tried multiple times to schedule scans, but our local hospital was not as advanced then as it is now and there were on-going problems with the equipment that kept delaying the scans. Finally in March they discovered it was cancer. Morris drove Steve to Lansdowne Hospital for tests on a Wednesday. The next Friday we brought dinner over to their house, along with the funniest movie we could think of, "The Gods Must Be Crazy," in an effort to cheer them up. The movie made Steve laugh out loud but laughing was painful for him and we had to cut it short. Steve had a rough night, and Ellen took him to Lansdowne hospital in the morning.

Steve's shortness of breath was caused by fluid buildup around his lungs. To get relief, the fluids had to be drained the same way I later had to have ascites drained. His doctors said he was too weak for chemo, but then some days later they ended up giving him a very strong dose of chemo anyway. He was never conscious again after that and the following Tuesday, May 4, 2010, Steve died. He first noticed symptoms in January and by May he was gone. We were devastated. It was intensely painful for his family, as well as for his relatives and friends. Steve was a young man of only 38.

Steve had a deadly form of cancer, Sarcoma, that generally strikes young men around his age, and is very fast growing and aggressive. Steve's wife, Ellen, does not blame the chemo for what happened to him. She says that it is such an aggressive and fast moving form of cancer that by the time Steve was diagnosed it had already spread like wildfire and was in his lungs and all throughout his body.

Steve and Ellen were scheduled to have their first appointment with a Sarcoma specialist in DC on the Monday after he was admitted to Lansdowne Hospital, but

Steve never made it to that appointment. They did not have time to try any other treatments. It was only a week and a half from the official diagnosis until he went into the hospital and two and a half weeks later he passed away.

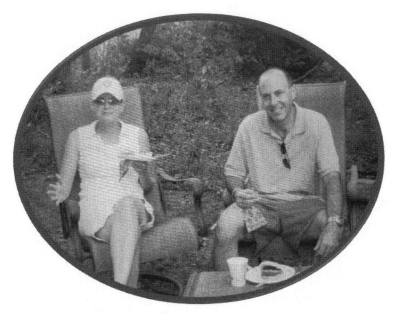

Steve and Ellen at an outdoor picnic at our house the summer before he passed away. Death is not something that only happens to the elderly. None of us know for certain how much time we have left.

The statistics for surviving Sarcoma are very dismal. One of Steve's doctors told Ellen that he had never seen anyone survive Sarcoma. He thought it might have been a blessing in disguise that it was diagnosed so late, because if they had found it earlier Steve would have gone through surgeries, amputations, treatments, etc. but most likely the outcome would have been the same.

Ellen has a good friend who lost her 9 year old daughter to the same type of Sarcoma. It started in the same part of her body and spread to her lungs as well. They caught it early and she went through many rounds of treatments and surgeries. The girl's family was very much into naturopathic treatments and healthy eating. They tried a combination of Naturopathic and Western Medicine, but they lost their daughter to Sarcoma just the same.

We were close to Steve and Ellen and we were extremely grieved by the entire experience. It made a huge impact on both Morris and I, and even now all these years later it still makes me tear up just thinking about it. It made us wonder what other treatments were available. There might not have been anything that could have been done for Steve, but even if that were true, was chemo the only option? If not, then what other options were there? I started to research, just as a personal interest and I found that there are many alternative treatments that have had good results. One therapy that came forward back then as most promising was the Gerson Therapy and I often talked to Morris about what I was learning.

DR. GARLAND

I first heard of Dr. Garland from my cousin, Linda. Her husband, Bruce had been told by his doctor that he had prostate cancer, and Bruce had turned to Dr. Garland for help. Dr. Garland had been a successful research analyst in Australia when he was diagnosed with a highly virulent form of cancer in his spine that had spread throughout his central nervous system. His doctors advised him to get his affairs in order, and told him he had no more than six months to live. There was nothing Western Medicine could do for him. Surgery and chemotherapy were not an option for his form of cancer, so instead of giving in to the doctors' diagnosis and giving up on life, he made a radical decision to quit his job and head off to India seeking answers.

In Australia, Ayurevedic medicine as practiced as it is in India, and it is held in high regard. He did not know what he would find in India, but he wanted to know what they were doing that he might be able to use to stay alive a little longer. Little did he know then that his search would take him all across India and Asia. All that happened over 30 years ago, so whatever he found worked for him after Western Medicine had completely failed.

Today he has a company selling vitamins and minerals for treating various conditions by supporting the immune system. I had a consultation with Dr. Garland by telephone. His approach to treating cancer also relied on diet, exercise, and supplements. He was familiar with the Gerson Therapy and approved of it, although his treatment was not identical. Being treated by Dr. Garland would require consultations by phone.

Dr. Garland's own battle with cancer perfectly demonstrates that Western Medicine is not the only valid form of health care in the world. Throughout human history and before the United States even existed, people have had to address health challenges. On every continent they have experimented with different treatments with varying degrees of success. Western Medicine did not cure Dr. Garland but 30 years after his terminal diagnosis he is still enjoying vibrant health.[2]

CANCER CENTER FOR HEALING

This clinic is located in Orange County, CA, not far from where we used to live. But now we live in Virginia and it is on the opposite side of the country, so it was not very accessible for long term treatment. Eventually we were able to visit the clinic. It's fairly large, and somewhat like a hospital, except patients don't stay there overnight.

They have a wide variety of treatments available such as;

- Insulin Potentiated Targeted Dose Chemo,
- High Dose Vitamin C Therapy,
- Hyperbaric Oxygen Therapy,
- Ozone Therapy,
- Far Infared Sauna Therapy,
- Personalized Nutritional Counseling,
- Nutraceuticals

These are only a small sample of their therapies; some are very cutting edge and even high tech, depending on what's needed. While we were initially trying to decide what to

---

[2] HTTP://WWW.BODYASDOCTOR.COM/WAYNE-GARLANDS-STORY

do, I called the clinic and had a consultation with one of their doctors by phone. It seemed like it might be a good place to be treated, but it would also be very costly. Since these treatments would not be covered by insurance and the clinic was so far away, it didn't seem like a realistic option for me.

COUSINS

Just a little before I was diagnosed with cancer, my Aunt Helen passed away and my cousin, Ken, emailed me to ask if I knew any historical family information for her obituary. I told him what I knew and that began a friendship between Ken and me (we had not spent any time together as children). Our friendship had just begun to bloom when I had to give him the bad news about my cancer diagnosis. Ken and his sister, Terrie, and brother, Tim, generously contributed toward my medical treatments which was so unexpected and extremely kind!

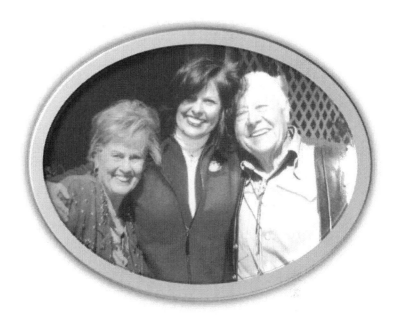

Aunt Helen (my mother's sister) and Uncle Obert;
their children are Ken, Terrie and Tim

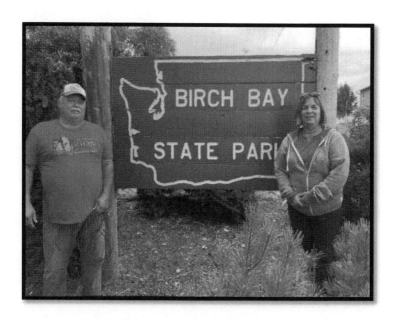

Cousin, Ken and his wife, Marsha

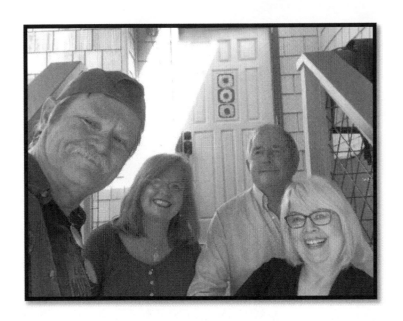

Cousin, Terrie and her husband David

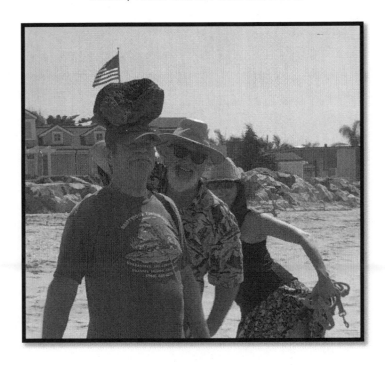

Cousin, Tim and his wife, Linda

INGER

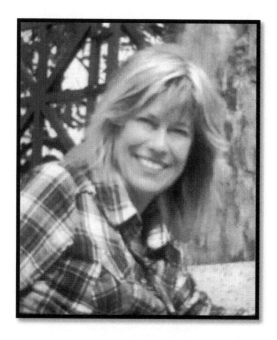

My cousin, Inger

My cousin, Inger, in Norway was aware that we really didn't have any local help from family, so she asked her supervisor if she could have leave to come help us. She was planning to fly all the way from Norway to the U.S. to be of assistance! She needed to clear it with us before making travel arrangements and though we would have dearly loved to see her, we decided it was really too much to ask. Even though we didn't take her up on her generous offer, we know she was sincere and she certainly would have come.

I'm not very sentimental or emotional, but the extravagant kindness of my extended family was overwhelming, and unforgettable. I am fortunate to have such caring cousins. I love them and I am very thankful for each of them!

What you find out when you are deathly ill is that the only thing that matters is the people you love and who love you. All the other stuff we spend a lot of time and energy on has no value at that point. People are what are important!

CHAPTER 2

STARTING THE PLAN

UTILITIES DEPARTMENT

While we were busy researching, I was also still working at the Utilities Department for the Town of Leesburg. It was a wonderful job with great medical insurance benefits and right then I needed those benefits more than ever. So I was apprehensive about telling anyone about my situation and possibly jeopardizing my job. On the other hand, I knew I couldn't conceal it indefinitely, and if I was struggling I felt I needed someone around who knew what was going on and could help me out if necessary. I just needed a little more time to think this through before making it public.

The person I knew the best at work, and trusted the most was my friend and coworker, Lesley. I asked her not to tell anyone and felt pretty confident that she would not because over the 6 years that I had known her I observed that she was good at keeping secrets. I suspect she took the news pretty hard. I'm just guessing on what happened next. Most likely her supervisor, John, caught her crying and probed and prodded until she finally told him. Then my secret slowly began to leak out.

Over the next days I began to suspect that other coworkers knew because of their atypical behavior. Ken put his arm around my shoulder as we walked down the hallway. He is my friend, but he never did that before! Herb stood watching me as I walked past so I asked him if he had heard something and he admitted he had. It became apparent that at least some people knew, but they were respecting my privacy.

It was probably silly and naive of me to think I could or even should keep it a secret for any length of time. I only did it for fear of endangering my job, or more importantly my medical insurance. When I finally told my supervisor, Sherry, she replied, "I'm glad you finally told me, because now I can start to put things into place that can help you." Obviously she was among those who already knew, and by trying to conceal my illness I was only slowing down implementation of programs that would be helpful to me.

When we finished talking about the business end of my illness Sherry asked, "How do you feel about all this?" I responded, "I am a Christian. If I get better, that's good. But if I die I go to heaven and that's good. So either way, I cannot lose." That was my honest reply, and that is why I had no fear from the very beginning when the nurse first informed me that I had ovarian cancer.

That answer probably startled her because she didn't know how to respond, but it was the truth. In the middle of the biggest health crisis of my life, I had perfect peace. I didn't like my situation, it wasn't fun. It was inconvenient, uncomfortable and difficult. But it wasn't frightening.

There are several things I learned through the experience and one of those is that I really do believe what I claim to believe. I don't just call myself a Christian. I truly believe that Jesus died for my sins, reconciling me to God so that I have perfect peace with Him. If I died I would have a place in heaven. If I did not die, well that's good too. I really couldn't lose, and I truly believe that. Observing my calm response to such terrible news proved it to me.

In the months to come I became extremely thankful for my job, my coworkers, my benefits and all the compassionate programs and support put in place for employees by the Town of Leesburg.

After all our research; talking to friends, medical and naturopathic doctors it was time to make a decision, and we chose the Gerson Therapy. The Gerson Therapy focuses on helping cancer patients strengthen their own immune systems to fight their disease, rather than relying on surgery, chemicals or radiation. As King David wrote, we are "fearfully and wonderfully made."[3] Our bodies are designed to heal and repair themselves. Helping the body to do what it was built for just made sense to us.

However, Gerson Therapy is not at all easy to practice. In fact now that I have had the experience of using the Gerson Therapy for five months as well as having two major surgeries and chemo; it's hard for me to decide which treatment was the most difficult. It was all hard!

Gerson Therapy is very demanding and requires training to be able to do it properly. It isn't an easy treatment to follow, but then neither is chemo. Dr. Amy had told me that I only had an 18% chance of success with chemo so it appeared to me that I wouldn't be any worse off trying something else. Morris called them to find out what I needed to do to be accepted.

---

[3] PSALM 139:14 (NLT)

Before I was diagnosed I had already been experiencing ascites, so fluids were accumulating in my abdomen with no way out. It is a very uncomfortable feeling, and the only relief is to have the fluids drained at a hospital. I had already had to have that done and four and a half liters were removed. Imagine how bloated you would feel with 4 ½ liters of fluid in your abdomen!

The Gerson Clinic accepted me, conditionally. They said they were not able to drain ascites so if it needed to be done I would have to leave the clinic and have it done elsewhere. Before coming to the clinic I had been gaining one liter of ascites per week. But they said that if I wanted to try we could come, and so we arranged to go to the Gerson Clinic in Tijuana, Mexico.

SOUTH OF THE BORDER

Having finally made a decision, we left for California on Monday, April 14, three and a half weeks after my initial diagnosis. Just before leaving for Mexico I wrote a letter to my coworkers. I asked Lesley to read to it to the men I worked with at the next weekly safety meeting. At that time the Utilities Department was largely comprised of men who installed and maintained the water and sewer lines, with only a handful of female office staff. They are all such great people! After hearing my letter, as a show of support they posed for a group photo wearing Minion goggles (like the cartoon, "Minions"). Lesley emailed it to me while we were in Tijuana and it brought a big smile to my face! They are all strong and tough men but at the same time kind and gentle.

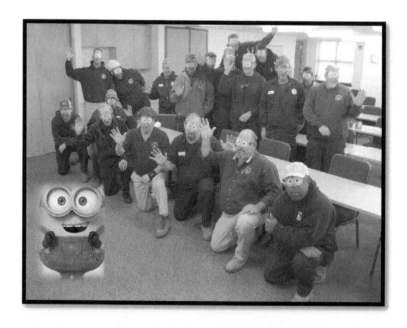

My coworkers after learning of my diagnosis and wearing Minion glasses; I love those guys!

We raised our family in Southern California and it was nice to have a little time to visit with family and friends including our son, Paul, and his family (Catherine, Carl and Ruby), my mom, and my sister, Lisa. Then we headed for the clinic in Mexico.

From the very beginning Morris was incredible. It was clear that he would do anything he could possibly do to help me get well. In fact, everyone was unbelievably kind and helpful. It seemed as if almost daily I was overcome by the latest random act of kindness. Daily we experienced outpourings of love and affection. I began saying "I love you" to everyone. People don't usually do that and neither do I ordinarily. It's a little awkward, but things change when you have cancer.

We all know we are going to die someday, but that day usually seems distant. When you have cancer you are confronted with the fact that that day might be much nearer than you thought. You don't want to miss any opportunity to show love or appreciation because you may not get another chance.

I think it made people feel a little awkward when I told them I loved them, and I understand that. I'd probably feel funny too, but I still figured that was better than wishing I had said something before it was too late. But that really is true for all of us, all the time. We have no control over many things that could happen to us, or to people we love. So we should always treat people as we would if it were to be the last time we'd see them.

Our pastor once said that he performs as many funerals for young people as he does for old people. The 16 year old daughter of a couple at the church, died when she crashed into a tree in the new car her parents gave her when she learned to drive. Another family at church had been at a family reunion where their 8 year old son enjoyed running and laughing with his cousins. Shortly after arriving home the boy died from an undiagnosed heart defect.

A 30 year old family man and neighbor on our street died when his three-wheeled motorcycle rolled over on him. Another time we were observers on a movie set. One young crew member in his 20's, was rushing equipment to the set and died when his Gator 4-Wheeler slid into a tree.

There was our friend, Steve; even though he was only 38 years old he died from cancer, and it happened fairly quickly. His wife, Ellen's, friend's daughter died of the same cancer at 9 years of age. Another of our friends had just sent his 19 year old son off to college where he died of an undiagnosed heart defect.

Just this morning as I write this, I learned that Jeff, the friend of a friend died a few days ago at the age of 27, leaving behind his girlfriend and 1 year old daughter. He had gone skateboarding without a helmet, fell, hit his head and died. My point is that young or old, none of us really knows how much time we have!

Our son, Paul, gave us a ride from Orange County to San Diego where we spent the night at a nice hotel arranged by the Gerson Clinic. In the morning we were picked up by a colorful fellow named "Jay" who chatted incessantly as he drove us across the border to the clinic in record time. We didn't have to show passports or even slow down. We just drove from San Diego past the long lines at the border, straight to the clinic without any delays.

Felix, the patient coordinator gave us a tour of the facilities and an orientation. Ines, a nurse took my blood and urine for labs. Then we had our first Gerson breakfast which is salt and sugar free, no meat or dairy, bland, tasteless and boring to be honest. I suppose I'm terrible to describe it like that because it was all very wholesome and healthy food, but I would be insincere if I said otherwise.

However, I chose not to do chemo so I was compelled to do the other hard thing (and it was very hard indeed, for me anyway). With the right spices the vegan food still might have been tasty but salt and spices are not part of the diet for whatever reason.

At breakfast we met Todd and Kim from Fredericksburg, Virginia, not far from where we live. Todd was suffering from stage IV melanoma and first sought treatment from a hospital specializing in melanoma. His doctors said that if Todd followed all their recommendations he had a 1% chance of recovery! One percent! That might as well be zero! Those odds were so bad that just about anything would be an improvement so he opted to go with the Gerson Therapy. Todd wore a sling on his right arm because the cancer was eating through the bone. His doctor warned that his arm was so fragile that it could break at any moment.

Melanoma is very difficult to treat and has an extremely low survival rate in advanced stages, but Todd has subsequently made a full recovery! Morris and I visited Todd at his home in Florida at the beginning of 2018 and he is in excellent health. He frequently goes scuba diving, his favorite sport. His incredible recovery speaks volumes about the efficacy of the Gerson Therapy.

Both the staff and the clients were very friendly and helpful. Because we were all in the same desperate situation we quickly formed a strong bond and were mutually supportive.

After breakfast we met Dr. Cervantes, who talked to us about the therapy and gave me a physical. Because I had ascites, Dr. Cervantes did not put me on as many juices as others were getting (10-13). His goal was to slow down the ascites, and maybe even have some of it reabsorb into my system. So I was to keep fluids to a minimum and I only received 6 juices a day. That was a tremendous relief to be honest because with all that fluid pressure caused by the ascites I really had no appetite. One requirement of the Gerson Therapy is that you must be able to eat. I was admitted on a day by day basis so what happened with those ascites would determine whether or not this was going to work for me.

Dr. Cervantes related a fascinating and encouraging account of one of his patients who was admitted with stage IV ovarian cancer with ascites, just like me. She already had 8 children when she was diagnosed and Dr. Cervantes advised her not to get pregnant, but she did get pregnant. He put her on the same regimen that I was on. He told us that as of the time we were talking to him the baby was 6 years old, and the mother was doing fine, no trace of cancer; very good news!

The Gerson clinic is located in Tijuana, Mexico, because it is not an approved treatment in the United States. One hears varying accounts of whether Tijuana is a safe place to be so that was a bit concerning. There were 2,506 killings reported in Tijuana in 2018 making it one of the most dangerous places in the world.[4] But the clinic and the surrounding area was quiet, pleasant, and felt very safe. It was situated not far from the beach and provided a tranquil setting so we could focus on healing.

The next day Dr. Cervantes reviewed my blood work and the results were encouraging. One goal of the therapy is to help patients become alkaline because that creates an unfavorable environment for cancer. Most Americans are

_____

[4] HTTPS://WWW.TRAVELTRIVIA.COM/MOST-DANGEROUS-CITIES/

acidic because of the type of foods we eat. Seven is neutral, and I was at 8 (alkaline!) so what Morris and I had been doing before we went there must have been at least partly right. None of our new friends were as alkaline as I was. Also, my kidneys and liver were in good shape which was very important if the Gerson Therapy was going to work for me.

I liked the doctors, staff, and all the people there. One friend, Pier, from San Francisco, said it felt like a sanctuary, and in a way it did. Everything was slow paced and relaxed. It had snowed in Virginia the night before but it was 64 in Tijuana and I sat in the sun soaking up that lovely warm feeling. There was a doctor and nurse on staff at all times so any questions were quickly answered and I felt very relaxed and happy to be there! I had such a good feeling about the place!

The following day the doctor measured my abdomen and it appeared that the ascites were decreasing and reabsorbing, which was very good news! Morris and I walked to the local Walmart, which was just about identical to one in the US, and then we walked down to the beach where we saw the big border wall separating the United States from Mexico.

People came to the clinic, literally from all over the world. One man came from Australia, a father and son came from Singapore. The father had nose cancer and had chemo therapy for it but it did not work. There was nothing more that Western Medicine could do for him so this was his last chance. Eric and Mary Elizabeth were from Maine. Atanas and his wife, Vasilka were from Eastern Europe. Vasilka had lung cancer and had received chemo therapy, which worked for a period of time but the cancer had returned. She had advanced ascites and the doctors had run out of options so she was trying Gerson. Maritza came from the Philippines. Some came because they felt it was their last chance, but for others like me the Gerson Therapy was their first choice.

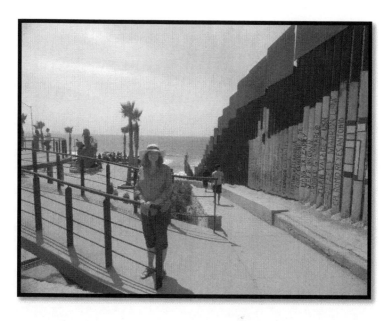

The border wall between Mexico and San Diego

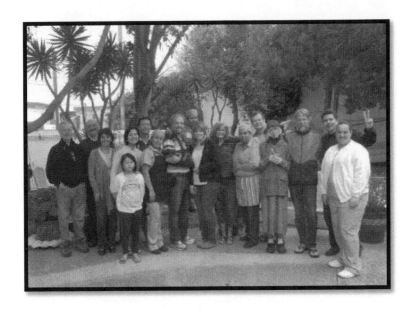

Group photo of people at the clinic while we were there

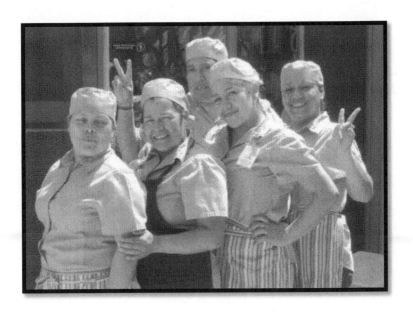

The kitchen staff

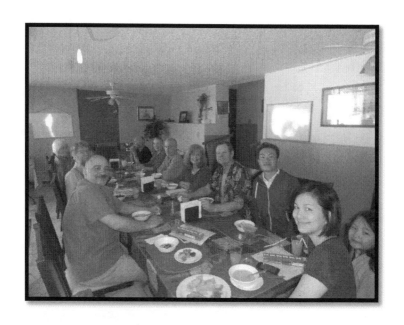

Group meals with the patients at the clinic were enjoyable
times of interesting conversations

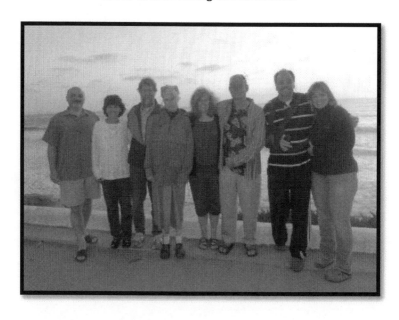

A group outing to the seaside

We met a Registered Nurse at the clinic named Mary Ann, who had administered chemo to patients for a number of years. She said that if she spilled even one drop of chemo on her skin she had to file an incident report (sort of like a Hazmat spill) because it is so toxic. But they would take that same toxic substance and drip it right into a patient's veins! Mary Ann got so tired of seeing patients die that she changed her vocation entirely. Most of the patients I spoke to who had already had chemo had discouraging things to say about it. Most of them regretted having chemo, or said that if it was helpful in diminishing their cancer, it did not go far enough.

Leaving the Gerson Clinic was bitter-sweet. It was so tranquil and harmonious there, and now we were heading back into the real world. Somehow we were going to have to make this program work without the helpful staff making the juices and meeting our needs. I had to go back to work and try to function like a normal employee, while battling a potentially terminal illness.

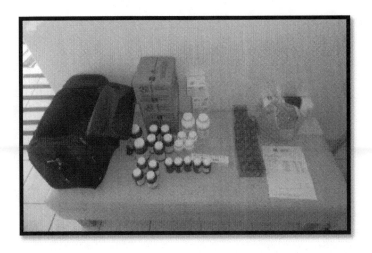

All the supplements we brought home from the clinic.

Our drive back across the border into the United States was as swift and uneventful as the ride into Mexico had been. Our friend, Bill, and our son, Paul, picked us up in San Diego, and we remained in Orange County for a couple more days, visiting friends and family. My sister, Lisa, allowed us to have a little party at her home so friends could visit with us. At that point no one knew if I would recover so there was the very real possibility that this would be the last time they would see me. Finally it was time to head home, get back to work and continue the Gerson Therapy on our own.

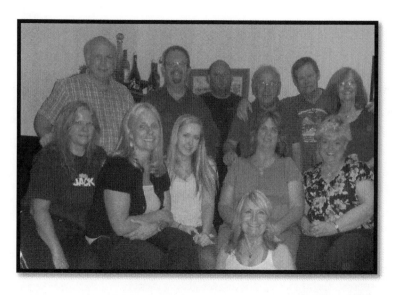

Some of our family and friends who visited
with us while in California

In some ways the Therapy is simple and non-invasive there are no medications to take, no cutting, burning, or poisoning (surgery, radiation or chemo). But on the other hand it is very labor intensive. There is so much involved

57

that Eric and Mary Elizabeth, and Todd and Kim remodeled their kitchens to simplify everything. It would be impossible to do it by myself without help; I would not even try.

The Gerson Therapy relies primarily on a diet of freshly juiced organic vegetables and fruits, oatmeal, potatoes, and a vegetable based soup called Hippocrates Soup, as well as other nutritional supplements. No one could ever get all the enzymes and nutrients available in 2 pounds of carrots by eating them because they have far too much bulk. One would have to chew ceaselessly and their stomach would be too full to finish them all. But it is easy to drink the juice from 2 pounds of carrots and benefit from all that condensed nutrition.

I love sweets and I expected that the most difficult part of the diet would be going without sugar, but I didn't miss sugar one bit. The one thing I missed terribly was salt. I don't know what the logic is for completely forbidding salt because the body requires some salt as an essential nutrient. In our culture we consume far too much salt, but we still need some salt.

Oatmeal, potatoes and soup without any salt or spices tastes bland, so it was always very difficult for me to get those foods down. I had such an aversion to them that I really thought that after I recovered I would never, ever, voluntarily eat them again. But later, once I could dress them up with salt and spices again I got over my aversion and didn't have a problem with them anymore.

I love to eat and have always had a good appetite (maybe too good) but by that time I didn't feel like eating at all. To be successful with the Gerson Therapy I had to eat.

Though the food was healthy, without salt it was tasteless and I didn't want to eat it, but I had to and eating was a daily struggle for me. I felt like the Salt Monster from the old original Star Trek TV series that had an overpowering craving for salt.

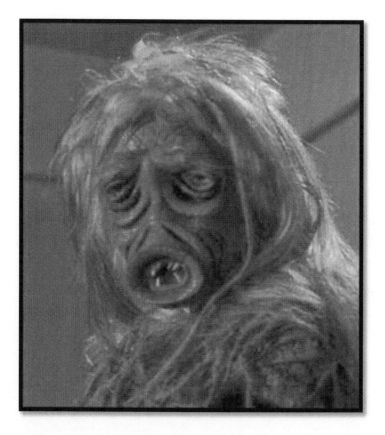

Star Trek Salt Monster

Another unpleasant aspect of the salt free diet was that almost every night without fail after struggling to get into bed, and finely getting comfortable, my feet would get strong painful cramps. That required me to quickly leap out of bed to stand on my feet to stretch out the cramps. I don't cry easily but this was such a frustrating and difficult ritual that it drove me to tears! Later when I discontinued the Gerson Therapy and began eating salt again, the cramps stopped immediately the very same day, and never returned.

As the weeks progressed, eating became increasingly problematic. In time I began to watch the clock in dismay as lunch time approached. I had always looked forward to lunch with my coworkers and the pleasant conversations that accompanied it, but having to force down that unappetizing food when I didn't feel like eating to begin with was a dreadful undertaking. I was always glad when lunch was over with; but then it would soon be time for dinner and the struggle would resume.

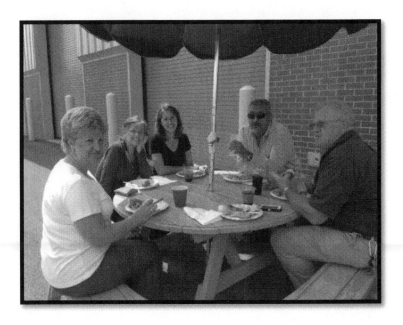

Lunch with a few of my coworkers, something I used to look forward to very much! Megan, Aref, Robert, and Lisa

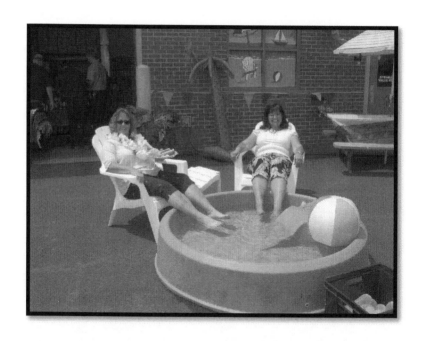

Lesley and I at the "Beach Party."
I had a lot of fun with my coworkers, especially at
lunch time; the best part of the job!

I had to get up around 5:00 AM every morning to make it to work on time, but Morris got up at 4:00 AM to prepare all the foods and juices I would need for the day. They had to be fresh, so they couldn't be prepared in bulk in advance; it had to be fresh every morning. It was a lot of work for Morris, but he never complained.

My acupuncture doctor noticed how attentive Morris was and observed, "He is very devoted, isn't he?" His dedication was obvious to everyone. Dr. Tuan said he had periodically seen husbands or wives desert their spouse during trying times with some absurd excuse like, "we'd get a tax break if we are apart, we can get back together later." But they never did get back together later.

In my opinion, abandoning a loved one when they are in such a weak and vulnerable state and are in urgent need of assistance is very dishonorable. I'm thankful that I could unquestioningly rely on Morris. I expected that and believed it to be true, but now it had been proven with certainty.

Morris made a mess of the kitchen though. The juicing and cooking he did was labor intensive, and there were jars and pans everywhere. He had a system and things were set up in a way that worked for him, and maybe I could not have done any better if I were in control. The kitchen wasn't dirty, but it was cluttered. I couldn't look at it, because there wasn't a single thing I could do about it. I barely had the energy to stand up and it felt abnormally difficult to walk so there was no way I could straighten things up. I'm not really sure why it was so hard to walk or even stand, because the muscles were all working, but I was so incredibly weak! I was very thankful that Morris was willing to do all that, and I know it was not easy to do.

Many friends wanted to help and asked about bringing meals but the Gerson diet is very specific. There were certain combinations of organic vegetables that needed to be prepared in a very exact manner. Because of that, no one could really help us with meals at that point. Instead many people gave us grocery store gift cards, and that helped so much because we were buying massive quantities of organic produce!

One highlight during that time was a visit from our longtime friend, Nelda. She was on her way from North Dakota to Turkey, but chose to detour to Virginia to visit us. That detour probably increased her fare by $1000 but it was such a kind and meaningful gesture. She may have thought she should see me while she still could, and there was very good reason to think that. Her visit in July 2014 was one of the bright spots in an otherwise difficult year.

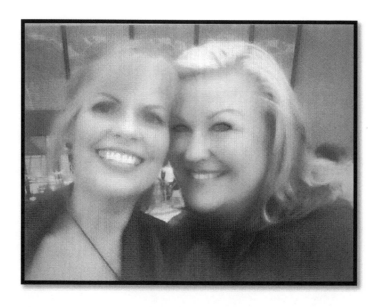

Carol and Donelda

GOING FROM BAD TO WORSE

My weight continued to plummet, which was why Dr. Belote had advised me to "Eat well." I worked very hard at eating well, but without an appetite, and with cancer robbing calories it was hard not to lose weight. By September of 2014 my weight was perilously low and I was in real trouble. Summer had passed and I remember driving home from work one evening and wondering if I would ever see summer again. I lay in bed one night wondering how much time I had left, and my intuitive guess was maybe a few more weeks.

One afternoon at work I had laboriously gotten my food and juices down, only to throw it up immediately. That was extremely discouraging because I didn't want to eat in the first place but I had managed to get it all down only to immediately lose all that effort. Fortunately I had been eating outside and Dave, a kind coworker, hooked a hose up to a fire hydrant and hosed off the asphalt. Everyone was so understanding and compassionate. I would soon learn why it was so hard to eat. Basically I could not eat, because my body was no longer able to process food.

My coworker, Ken, overheard me telling my office companion, Lisa, that none of my clothes fit anymore. With so much weight loss I was down 4 sizes and most of my clothes hung on me like a tent. The next day Ken brought in numerous bags of clothing that his wife wasn't using. They were mostly size 8 or 10 and they all fit me perfectly. Many of them were brand new! I love clothes so it was fun sorting through it all.

My good friend, Ellen, also brought some new clothes over. She has good taste and I loved the things she brought. These surprising expressions of care and concern made being ill bearable and sometimes even uplifting.

As I lost weight I also grew weaker; life was gradually draining away and I could feel it. I tried my best to look good each day, but I was losing so much weight that I didn't have much more to spare. I'm sure my coworkers were in doubt that I would make it. I know for certain that

I was in doubt! I was so thin that I had to sleep with a pillow between my legs so the bones didn't rub against each other!

Knowing that my time on earth might be quickly coming to an end, the last place I wanted to be was sitting in an office. I wanted to be outside or spending time with my family and friends, not tied to a desk. One time a well-meaning coworker, Ozzy, whose father had died of cancer a couple years before came to my office and asked me, "What are you doing here? You know how this is going to end. Why are you wasting your time here?" I can assure you that I agreed with him wholeheartedly and had often thought the same thing, but I needed medical insurance, so I needed that job.

Another time my coworker, Terry, told me that he thought I was doing the right thing by not taking the chemo route. He had firsthand experience with ovarian cancer because his wife had it. He was reluctant to tell me how she was doing because sadly, she succumbed to it. She had chemo which only increased her pain and discomfort, and she died anyway.

Another coworker, Connie, said her sister had chemo. It was supposed to prolong her life by many months, but it did not give her much extra time at all. However, it did cause her a lot of extra suffering from the side effects so that what little time she had left became even more miserable.

I continued to hear discouraging firsthand accounts about chemo, and I didn't want to have it. I only heard one positive account from anyone, and that was Shawn.

Dr. Cervantez, my doctor at the Gerson Clinic, continued to monitor my progress. Each month I had a blood test taken and the results were sent to him. He'd review the results with me by phone, sometimes making positive comments, other times not so much. Now that I was having so much difficulty eating, my lab results were not as good. Eventually he consulted with the other 3 doctors on staff at the Gerson Clinic and they recommended that I try chemo! Chemo? What?! Dr. Cervantes said that he didn't like it either but I was going downhill fast and they did not know what else to try.

Charlotte Gerson, daughter of the founder, Dr. Max Gerson, often forcefully and emphatically declared that "Chemo does not work! It does not work!" And now the doctors from that very same clinic were recommending chemo to me!

If Charlotte Gerson's statement was correct and chemo does not work, then why were they recommending it? To me that suggested that they were grasping at straws. Gerson Therapy was not going to work for me, so I should make one last, desperate, futile treatment attempt and try chemo (which according to Charlotte Gerson, was not going to work). It was obvious that we were going to have to stop the Gerson Therapy and take another direction. But now what? Time was running out.

It's very common for women with ovarian cancer to feel full even before eating and to have trouble with vomiting and shortness of breath, at least in part caused by the ascites. I learned that we all have fluid cycling through our abdomens to lubricate our organs. But it's not there all at once; it keeps cycling through and is reabsorbed.

With late stage ovarian cancer the cancer itself causes additional fluids to be generated, and the cancer also obstructs the places that would help to reabsorb the fluid. The fluids press against the organs making it hard for the stomach to expand when eating. It also presses on the diaphragm and can even move up around the lungs to press on them, making it harder to breath.

Once people have gotten to the point that they have ascites, the average survival time is 20 to 58 weeks. By this time I was at 25 weeks or more. The 4th time I had the fluid drained they removed 3.7 liters. I was relieved to get all that fluid out of there; it felt like I was 9 months pregnant. But it was disturbing that so much had accumulated so quickly.

My doctor said it's hard to get enough calories when you have cancer because the cancer is also competing for the calories so keeping my weight up was a big deal and I was doing very poorly in that department. I was also getting increasingly low on energy, at least partly due to a lack of nutrition.

The cancer had metastasized, meaning it had spread and was not in just one location. I usually envision this as a dandelion flower. If you could pick the flower before the seeds blow away you have an excellent chance of preventing hundreds of weed seeds from dispersing. But once the seeds blow off into the wind they go everywhere and you could never, ever collect them all.

In early stages of cancer it is all in one small location. If the cancer is discovered then the chances of preventing it from growing and spreading are good. But once the cancer cells have escaped from the original location and traveled to other parts of the body (metastasized) it's impossible to find them all again. That's why doctors never say cancer is 'cured'. They use the term 'remission' which means the cancer has subsided and at the present time there are no signs or symptoms of cancer. Remission can be temporary or permanent.

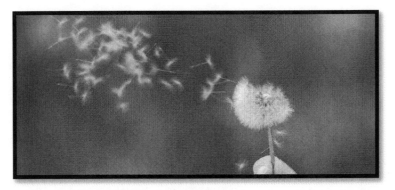

Dandelion seeds blowing away in the wind

Since my cancer was discovered after it had metastasized, the cancer cells had spread along the surface of the intestines leading to sores that created scar tissue that bound together the loops of the intestines, sort of like tying them up with string. This made it harder for the intestinal muscles to contract and propel contents along.

If nothing was done about it eventually it would lead to a complete bowel obstruction, meaning nothing would get through. This type of obstruction causes death in the majority of women who die of ovarian cancer and is partly why they are likely to starve to death. On the one hand I like to understand what is happening, why it's happening, and what to expect. But on the other hand, all the information I acquired was such bad news!!! From what I read, my oncologist, Dr. Amy, was right when she told me at the beginning that this is incurable. It was doubtful that either traditional or naturopathic medicine could do me much good.

When I first found out I had cancer we just went where the people at the emergency room made us an appointment. We didn't choose the oncologist and we didn't know her. I don't know why it took us so long to think of this, but we already knew a great oncologist.

Eleven years earlier, when we moved to Virginia, Morris's mom and dad drove out from Washington State to see our new home. Morris's father had a blood test just before they started driving east, and the doctor called him when they had reached Idaho to tell him that he should either turn around and head home or go straight to an oncologist when he arrived at his destination.

So when they arrived at our house I made an appointment for him with an oncologist named Dr. Rajendra, who we did not know at the time. He discovered that my father-in-law, Morris Sr., had leukemia! That was terrible news! He passed away about a year later, but we had all been very pleased by the excellent care Dr. Rajendra gave him. Now that we were finished with Gerson we went to see Dr. Rajendra for a second opinion.

Meanwhile, my naturopathic doctor, Dr. Stewart, called Dr. Cervantez to collaborate with him and we came away with a few helpful suggestions. From the beginning I had strongly wanted to avoid chemo, not because I didn't think it works but because of the massive collateral damage it does. Dr. Stewart told us about another form of chemo (Insulin Potentiated Chemo) that uses only 1/10th as much but is still very effective.

I was still not thrilled about this, but the ascites were building up too quickly and it was time for more drastic measures. So we planned to look into it, along with Vitamin C IV's. He also recommended for the second time an acupuncturist, Dr. Tuan. Dr. Stewart said Dr. Tuan was very good at assisting the lymphatic system. My lymph glands were clogged up by the cancer which is one reason why the ascites were not draining and Dr. Stewart thought Dr. Tuan could be a great deal of help with that. So we finally made an appointment with him. I really wish we had seen him when Dr. Stewart first told us about him, but better late than never.

Only 12 days after the previous paracentesis I had to have the ascites drained again and they removed 3.5 liters of liquid protein. Obviously, this was very bad news.

I asked Morris to pray for me that night. Part of his prayer was, "God, please don't take my wife" and I broke down. I have many people that I love dearly and many people love me in return. I didn't feel like I was finished here yet, but by now if I was going to survive I would need nothing short of a miracle, nothing less would do. Reality can be very cruel.

Right in the middle of all this turmoil, Morris and I celebrated our 40th wedding anniversary. When he promised, 'for better or for worse' he couldn't have foreseen this horrendous ordeal, but Morris stood by me though all of it, doing absolutely everything he could do to support me and help me heal.

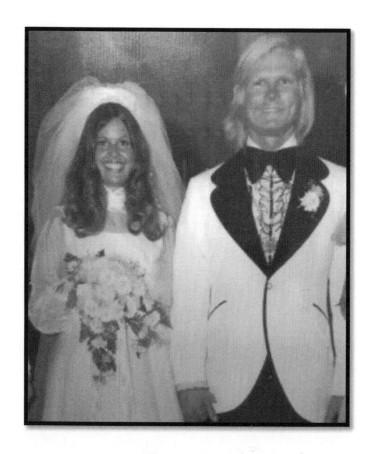

Our wedding day

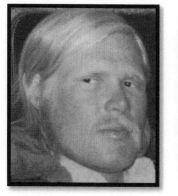 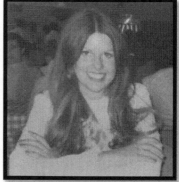

Carol and Morris while dating

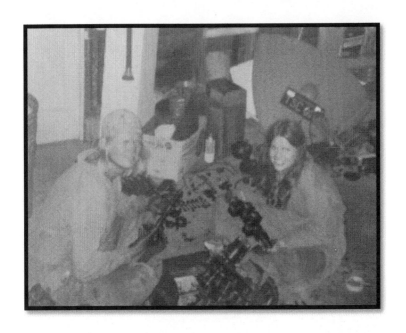

Rebuilding my old VW

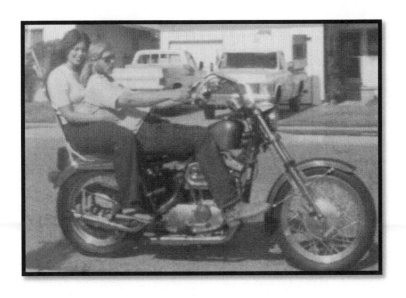

Morris's Harley Davidson Motorcycle
(He sold it so we could take a 3 week honeymoon in Europe!)

CHAPTER 3

CHANGE OF PLANS

allopathic medicine;
> *A system in which medical doctors and other healthcare professionals (such as nurses, pharmacists, and therapists) treat symptoms and diseases using drugs, radiation, or surgery. Also called, conventional medicine, mainstream medicine, and Western medicine.* [5]

Now we were making a sharp change of direction, from naturopathic to allopathic medicine and we met with my new oncologist, Dr. Ragendra. He has been featured in many magazines such as "Top Doc" and that is understandable. We felt much more at ease with him. I learned from one of the techs at the hospital that Dr. Rajendra and his family support and operate an orphanage in India, which speaks volumes about his character. He is a very gentle and pleasant man who listened very carefully to what we had to say.

We told him that we had gone to the Gerson clinic and he said he had other patients who had gone there as well. Looking at my labs he repeated at least three times, "I have to say I'm very impressed." My lab results were much better than he would have expected at that advanced stage of my illness. He said it could be attributed to my otherwise strong and healthy biological make-up, or to the

---

[5] HTTPS://QUIZLET.COM/183850698/COMPLEMENTARY-ALTERNATIVE-THERAPIES-FLASH-CARDS/

Gerson Therapy. He said an argument could be made either way.

We asked Dr. Rajendra if surgery might be advisable to remove as much of the cancer as is possible. He said it is difficult to find surgeons willing to perform surgery without first having chemo, but he knew a surgeon at MedStar Hospital in Washington, D.C. who he thought might be willing to try, Dr. Mark Steves. We made an appointment with him for the following Tuesday.

By now my health was in steep decline so our son, Paul, came for a visit from California (for all we knew this could be his last visit with me still living) and he brought along our grandson, Carl. I was in such bad shape by then that we did not think we could handle a baby around so sadly Paul's wife, Catherine and our granddaughter, Ruby, stayed at home. I had a couple of doctor appointments scheduled during their visit which was very disappointing to me because I wanted to spend every single moment enjoying their company, not visiting doctors. But the ascites were getting worse and we needed to act quickly.

I had only been in the hospital twice in my life and that was to have babies. I was not looking forward to having major surgery, but at least we had a direction. In the meantime I planned to enjoy the company of Paul and Carl as much as possible and try to forget for at least a little while that I was a cancer patient in very bad shape.

We took a family trip to the zoo, a brief walk on the Washington and Old Dominion Trail, and did a little sightseeing in Washington, D.C. on the day of my appointment with my surgeon. I always rode in a wheelchair, not because I couldn't walk, but because it was very difficult to walk or stand for long. In a wheelchair I could just ride and enjoy the activities

74

without being quickly worn out. Whenever we went shopping I rode around in those motorized shopping carts. It felt strange, but it was that or I couldn't go anywhere, I just couldn't walk.

As if we didn't have enough on our plate, on September 3rd we learned that Morris's aging mother in Washington State had a major stroke and was not expected to live much longer. That would be bad news at any time, but especially bad timing as I was about to have major surgery.

My oncologist, Dr. Rajendra, put in a good word for me which was how we were able to get an appointment with Dr. Steves so quickly. Dr. Steves told us that each time I had the ascites drained it was 'a huge protein loss.' It might make me feel better for a little while by relieving the pressure, but each time I did it I was going farther downhill. The last time they drained the ascites they withdrew 5 liters! That's about 1 1/3 gallons, so I had been very uncomfortable!

Dr. Steves said that surgery to remove as much cancer as possible would help slow down the ascites. He would not be able to get it all so he still recommended chemo, though he did not insist upon it as a condition for doing the surgery. But even if the surgery went well it would not be a solution. In Dr. Steves' words, "it will only keep you on the planet a little while longer." Just before leaving the office he turned back, looked directly at me and said, "You know you're going downhill, don't you?" I guess that was his way of making sure I was aware of just how bad my situation was. We would all soon discover that I was in much worse condition than any of us had imagined!

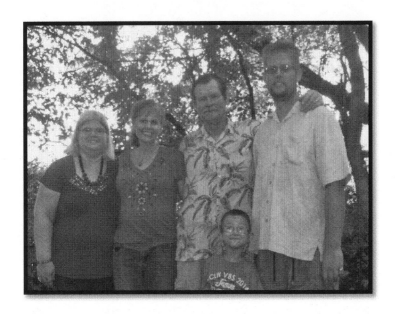

Our daughter, Crystal, Carol, Morris, our grandson, Carl and son, Paul taking a short walk on the Washington and Old Dominion Trail

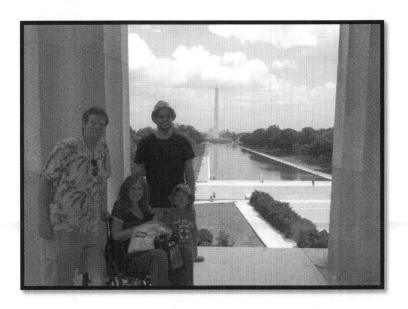

In Washington D.C. to meet my surgeon, Dr. Steves

Because I had always enjoyed excellent health and had no other risk factors like high blood pressure or diabetes, Dr. Steves thought I would be a suitable candidate for surgery. Dr. Ragendra and Dr.Steves both respected my desire to avoid chemo although they both recommended it, and I really appreciated that. Dr. Steves told me to get a CAT scan by the end of the week, and he could do the surgery the following week. We were astonished by how quickly he was moving things along, but Dr. Steves said he wanted to do the surgery as soon as possible to avoid having another ascites drain and the additional protein loss.

The surgery would be at MedStar Hospital in Washington, D.C., and we were told to expect to be in the hospital for 5-6 days; possibly more if the colon or intestines were involved. The surgery would last between 4 to 8 hours depending on how well my vital signs held up. He said he would try to get me a private room so Morris could stay in the room with me.

We have always tended to have *major* life events occur in August and slightly into September so every year we joke about what it's going to be this time. We made it through August so we thought we were in the clear, but a few days into September we were facing the ordeal of major surgery along with Morris's mother's stroke. Life sure can be hard, and just when we thought it couldn't get any harder, it did!

To spare us the long drive to Washington, D.C. to deliver my CAT scan and EKG results, Dr. Steves' arranged to have his assistant, Belinda, meet us at a local Starbucks to hand off the results. We thought she would hurry in and out, but to our surprise she chatted with us for an hour and 15 minutes! She answered all our questions and made us feel very much at ease.

Then we went shopping for 'normal' food for the first time in over 5 months. I had been a vegetarian for 5 full months, and to be really honest, I hated every minute of it. I wish I could say it was great, but I would be lying. The complete lack of seasonings was the main reason it was so disagreeable. It's possible I might not have hated being a vegetarian if I could spice things up a bit because I do have some vegetarian dishes that I prepare and enjoy.

But switching back to 'normal' food wasn't easy either. Normal food tasted very foreign and it was uncomfortable to eat it. That evening we went to "On the Border" Mexican Restaurant to get fajitas, something I had been craving for months. They tasted outstanding, but in spite of that I didn't feel like eating, which was scary. Now that I could eat anything, I still didn't want to eat. There was the hope that after surgery there would be less ascites and more room for food so maybe food would be more appealing.

It's kind of hard to believe looking back, but while all of this was going on I was still working a regular full time work week! I had to take time off for doctor appointments, but I was trying to conserve my leave not knowing how much time would be spent recuperating from surgery, or getting other doctor treatments.

On September 9, 2014 after a light breakfast I headed off to work as usual. My coworkers were encouraging and supportive as always. My friend, "Hillbilly," made a special point of sitting with me during lunch break and even wrote a little poem for me. I expected to have surgery and return to work in a few weeks, not knowing at the time that would be my last day actually working for the Town of Leesburg.

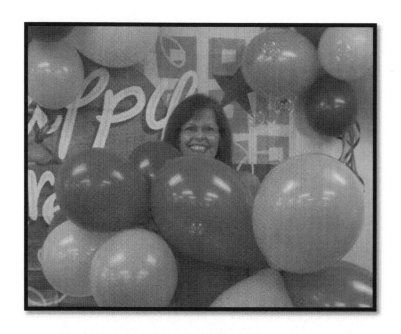

My last day working in the Utilities Department; the day before my first major surgery. The festive photo was taken to celebrate the retirement of the Town Manager.

Morris picked me up from work a little after lunch and we spent the night at a hotel near the hospital to make sure that traffic would not cause us to be late. The surgery was scheduled for September 10th at 11:30 AM. After the long hospital intake process they finally wheeled me down the hall to the operating room.

There was a big fish eye mirror in the hallway so I could see behind me into the waiting room as they wheeled me away. Morris was standing there with a concerned expression, trying to catch one last glimpse of me as I was being wheeled out of sight and he was forced to trust me to the care of others. That is an image forever burned into my memory.

MY FIRST MAJOR SURGERY

The clean, white tiled walls of the operating room were lined with numerous large containers filled with every imaginable shape of pointed and sharp implements. Five nurses were busily preparing the operating room for the surgeon. They each introduced themselves and that was the last thing I knew. The anesthesiologist did not tell me when he administered the anesthesia, and I was unconscious before I even knew what happened. The next thing I was aware of was waking up in the recovery room with an unbearable sense of thirst.

I had not had anything to drink since midnight the day before the surgery and I woke up in the recovery room under a nurse's watchful care with an agonizing desire for water. That was the most thirst I have ever experienced, and at that point my all-consuming thought was water. I wasn't in any actual danger of becoming dehydrated because I was hooked up to an IV drip, but I hadn't thought of that and my throat and mouth felt incredibly dry. My sensation of extreme dehydration was mostly psychological, but that did not diminish my desperation for water one bit.

In many ways the surgery itself was much more painful for Morris than it was for me, because I was asleep and unaware of what was happening around me. Shortly after the surgery began, two of our closest friends, Ellen and Paula, arrived at the hospital to wait with Morris during the 6 hour surgery. They all decided to head for the cafeteria to get some lunch, and had barely gotten seated, when an announcement came over the loudspeaker that "Morris Nylander should return to the waiting room." Morris was directed to a tiny room where he waited 15-20 minutes to talk to Dr. Steves.

Dr. Steves had only just begun the surgery and half an hour into it he decided to wash up and talk to Morris before continuing. Dr. Steves told Morris, "I have bad news, and more bad news." It looked very much worse than what the CAT scans revealed. He found that the cancer was extremely advanced; "it was "everywhere." The cancer had fused to most of my organs so that he was unable to do the planned hysterectomy. There wasn't much he could remove without damaging critical organs. He said most surgeons would have sewn me up right then, which would have meant it was all over for me, but he opted to discuss it with Morris first.

Fortunately the hospital made it very easy to set up an Advance Directive, which made it possible for me to designate someone else to make medical decisions as my representative in case I was unable to do so, and of course I designated Morris. If I had not had an Advanced Directive the doctor would most likely have ended the surgery at this point.

Dr. Steves told Morris that I had been starving because the cancer had permeated and blocked my intestines. My intestines could no longer process food and without radical intervention I would have certainly died of starvation within 2-3 weeks. That explained why over the last few weeks I had noticed my strength was decreasing at a much faster pace.

The only remaining option left was for Dr. Steves to remove the parts of the intestines that were blocked by cancer so that I could at least process food again, but this would require a colostomy. Morris did not really know what a colostomy was (neither did I at that point), but he told the surgeon to proceed.

A colostomy is a surgical operation in which a piece of the colon is diverted to an artificial opening in the abdominal wall so as to bypass the damaged part of the colon. The part of the colon that comes through the abdominal wall is called a stoma. The stoma serves the same purpose as the anus. Fecal matter would no longer pass through the anus, but out of the stoma so a bag would be required to capture waste. The bag had a hole to surround the stoma and was attached to the skin around the stoma by a strong adhesive. The bag was completely open at the bottom so waste could be drained out when sitting on the toilet, and a removable clip sealed it closed when finished.

The same bag can be used for several days then needs to be replaced with a new bag. If the seal around the stoma is anything less than perfect the skin around it can become sore and inflamed but the bag must still be worn at all times, no matter how irritated and sore the skin may become. There are a wide variety of seals, powders, gels, etc. designed to improve the seal around the stoma and they help, but no matter what you do you can't consistently get an absolutely perfect seal.

The bags have a limited capacity; gassiness can also inflate and fill the bag. The bag needs to be emptied before it becomes overfull or it could push away from the skin and empty all over everything (thankfully that never happened to me!)

A colostomy is a very nasty thing, but if the alternative is death it's the best option available. Morris made the right decision, and the one I would have made for myself. Otherwise I would have had to recover from surgery without having received any positive benefit from it at all.

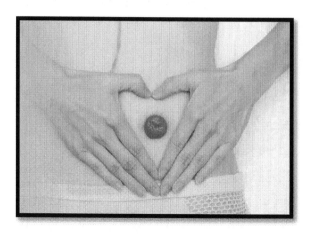

Example of a stoma; a portion of the intestines that comes through the abdominal wall

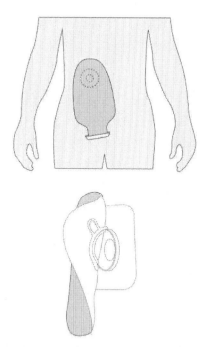

Colostomy bag covers the stoma to collect waste, and is emptied at the bottom from an opening with a removable clip.

Morris authorized Dr. Steves to proceed and walked back to the cafeteria where Paula and Ellen were waiting. They were anxious to hear what the doctor said, but Morris was unable to speak. He had just been told that the cancer was everywhere and basically there wasn't anything the doctor could do about it. A colostomy would allow me to eat and process food, but that is all, it didn't do anything to reduce the cancer. It sounded like a death sentence and Morris struggled hard to control his emotions.

Morris suggested to Paula and Ellen that they should all go outside and walk around a bit, thinking that might help him relax. The three of them were heading down the crowded cafeteria hallway when in the distance Morris saw his former coworker and good friend, Dave Charlton walking towards them from the other end of the hallway. Dave's arrival was completely unexpected, and perfectly timed; immediately after Morris had received that devastating news.

Dave said he had been at home working and felt the strong impression that God was telling him to "get up and go to the hospital, right now". I had posted information about my upcoming surgery on Facebook and Caring Bridge, but that is the only way Dave knew about it. He stopped working and left for the hospital immediately; arriving exactly after Morris received that devastating news.

MedStar Hospital is an enormous facility! I was still in surgery and did not have a room yet so if Dave had not been walking down the hall at that exact moment it would have been nearly impossible to locate Morris. Ellen, Paula and Dave spent the entire day with Morris and he needed their support so desperately; they were literally a 'godsend'. I would venture to say that was the most stressful and difficult day of Morris' life and their companionship helped to make the unbearable, a little more tolerable.

In the coming weeks Morris assumed that I was not going to live and his goal was to make life as comfortable and pleasant for me as possible for as long as he could. I'm pretty certain that nobody who had a complete and accurate understanding of my condition expected me to survive at that point.

RECOVERY

Morris's experiences throughout the surgical ordeal were horrible, but mine were not easy either. I woke up in the recovery room with a tube down my nose and that unbearable sense of thirst. One good thing throughout all of this was that outside of having cancer, I am a very strong and healthy person. They said my vital signs were 'like a rock' and so they did not need to send me to ICU as they did with most people. However I got a very rough start in the recovery room because whoever put the gastric nasal tube down my nose and throat made a small mistake and left it coiled 3 times inside my mouth.

The coils created the sensation that I was choking and if I tried to adjust the tube that sensation was strongly amplified. My mouth had never been drier in my life. It was dry to the point of painful but when after much pleading I was given ice chips, I could not swallow them without gagging and choking because of the coils in my mouth! That simple medical error alone caused me more pain and distress in the first night and day than anything else! They tried giving me lozenges, sprays, everything they could think of except no one thought of looking into my mouth! I didn't think to ask about it because for all I knew the coils were supposed to be there; I had never had surgery before and didn't know what was normal! At 3:00AM a private room became available and so Morris and I got to move upstairs. The room had a chair that folded into a bed for Morris, which was a huge help.

I was so preoccupied by that miserable tube that I wasn't asking any questions for which Morris was very grateful. He had been dreading having to tell me how advanced the cancer was, and that I now had a colostomy. His experience earlier in the day of being unable to speak is what caused him such anxiety. He didn't want to freeze up and scare me.

When he finally did tell me I wasn't really any more upset about the colostomy than I had been about being informed about having cancer in the first place. It's unpleasant, but there wasn't anything that could be done about it. What would have really upset me is if Dr. Steves had begun the surgery and closed me up without doing anything. Then I would still have to recover without any benefit at all from the surgery and I would not have been alive much longer. I would have certainly died from starvation.

Finally we got to talk to Dr. Steves briefly. He did not give us any additional information but he was perplexed about why the tube in my nose was bothering me so much. He remarked that the tube didn't look right. He had the technician check it and she was startled to discover the coils. She looked extremely disturbed while correcting it. That simple act of removing the coils in my mouth gave me instantaneous relief. But it was too late, the damage had already been done; my throat was very sore. My voice was reduced to a whisper and it did not completely return to normal for several months.

There was a cord attached to my bed with a green button on it that I could press every 6 minutes to self-administer a dose of Fentanyl to relieve pain. The logic is that patients feel less stressed when they have a degree of control over pain management. It worked well on pain, but I have a high tolerance to pain and didn't really need it much for that. The coils in my mouth may have been gone but I still had a tube down my nose and throat and that disturbed me more than anything else. Pain medication was no help at all in relieving that discomfort.

Our friend, Joe Njoku, came to visit Friday evening and brought a balloon and a lovely flower arrangement. Coincidently, Joe's sister works at MedStar hospital and she had come to my room earlier that day to offer to help us in any way she could, which was much appreciated.

Around this same time we received an update on how Morris's mom was doing, and it was not good news. Ordinarily, Morris would have flown to Washington immediately (and I would have gone with him if I wasn't so sick). But I was recovering from major surgery, and at that point it did not look likely that I would be alive much longer. Our good friend, Ellen, kindly offered to stay with me so Morris could go to see his mother one last time, but he just couldn't bring himself to leave me at that critical point in time. He just couldn't go.

I have no complaints about the care I received at MedStar, in fact I wrote a letter giving positive feedback for my nurses after I was released from the hospital. But nurses care for multiple people and they aren't able to respond immediately to every need. Though they are very careful, mistakes still happen, like the tube that was coiled in my mouth. I know Ellen would watch out for me, and I'm confident she would do an excellent job, but it would have been too stressful for Morris to leave just then and have to constantly wonder if I was alright.

Morris had to leave the hospital briefly to take care of some business at home in the morning so he missed the moment when my room was temporarily crowded with an entourage of 10 doctors. My surgeon directed all his comments to the other doctors, not to me. It was as if I was not even in the room! The only bit of information I gleaned from that visit was when Dr. Steves remarked to the other doctors that my 'bladder was unrecognizable' because the cancer was so prolific, which of course was not good to hear.

Our daughter, Crystal, and friend, Andrea also came to visit on Friday with cards, flowers and cheerful, smiling faces that helped to distract me from this steady stream of appalling news. I have a good relationship with Crystal so obviously this was hard for both of us. It was hard for me to know that my illness was the cause of so much suffering for people I love, but we got to affirm each other and I thought she would be alright.

In the afternoon I took a walk around the hospital floor with Morris and our nurse, Brittany. The nurses told me that the fastest way to get my intestines working so I could go home was to walk. So I walked a lot, much more than they required because I wanted to get out of there, fast!

On Sunday, I was greatly amazed by the stream of visitors that came to see me. Beginning around 1:00PM and ending at 10:30PM a steady stream of 8 people came to visit. I never expected anyone, not one, to come because it was such a long and miserable drive to the hospital. But it was refreshing and very touching. It helped to take my mind off my surroundings for a little while at least.

In summary, my surgery was a complete failure in the respect that the cancer was too far advanced for any of it to be removed as we had hoped. I did get a respite in having the cancerous parts of the intestine removed (60% of my large intestines and 40% of my small intestines) so that I was unlikely to starve to death in the next few weeks. So in that respect it wasn't a complete loss.

I had a colostomy then, something I was not very pleased about, but it was still better than facing imminent starvation. In every conceivable way, my situation appeared to be desperate and hopeless. Caring Bridge is a website that makes it easy for patients to keep friends and relatives informed with up to date information about their condition. This is what I wrote at that time on my Caring Bridge page about all this bad news;

> "I would like to say, that we have not given up. Things don't look good. In fact they almost could not look any worse than they do right now. However God has numbered my days before there were any of them. He knows how many hairs are on my head and has counted all my tears and kept them in a bottle. He is all knowing and all powerful. I know I have multitudes of people praying for me, they tell me so all the time. We still intend to look into any other possible life saving man made measures, but above all we are looking to the Great Physician. No one can keep me here if He wants to take me home, but nothing can take me out if He wants to keep me here either!"

It's hard going through something as difficult as cancer, but I cannot begin to imagine how much more difficult (unbearable really) it would have been without my faith in God; my Lord Jesus Christ. If I got better, that would be great. But if I did not get better I would go to heaven. That gave me 'peace that passes understanding' in the middle of profound misery.

Particularly difficult for me was that awful tube down the nose and throat because it caused a sharp soreness in my throat making it very hard to talk and it woke me up multiple times each night with searing pain. Ice chips were my best friends and only relief. Another struggle was resisting the temptation to panic and rip the tube out. I hyperventilated one night and I think it was caused by having that foreign object in my throat. Finally on September 15, the doctor and his entourage came in to tell me that they thought it was OK to remove the tube! Relief! Bliss! Joy! Happiness!

Once the tube was removed I felt an immediate sense of relief! They said they might start feeding me the next day but had to take it easy. Of course I had been losing weight for months and I was still not eating. But they didn't want me to become nauseous and start vomiting.

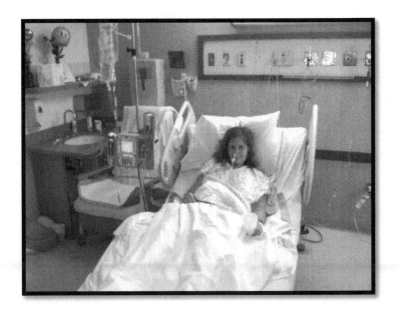

Carol in the hospital with the dreadful 'tube'.

Just 5 minutes after they removed the tube out of my nose

and throat, Morris' sister, Becky, called in tears to let him know that his mother had just passed away. I am certain that the Wednesday during my surgery was the hardest day of Morris' life, and the whole week had been trying. It's very hard to watch someone you love suffer and be powerless to do anything about it. And then his mother passed away at about the same time. Morris would have certainly gone to Washington for the funeral, but he couldn't possibly go while I was stuck in the hospital. Life was hammering him; one blow was followed by another.

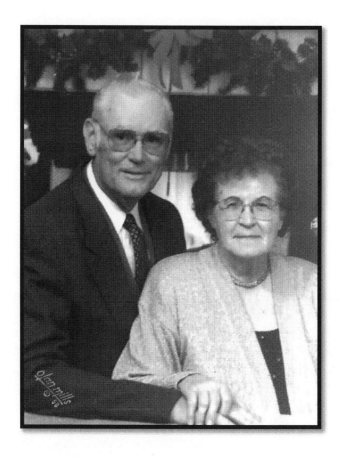

Morris's parents; Morris Sr. and LaVerne

My surgeon said I would have only lasted a few more weeks before starving to death and I believe it. Shortly before the surgery I laid in bed wondering how much more time I had left and guessed that I had a few more weeks. The entire time I'd been in the hospital they had not fed me, except whatever was in the IV drip, and that may have amplified my weakness. As a person who has always been strong and healthy it was hard to take feeling so weak. I often wondered if it would have been easier psychologically to accept being so feeble if I had struggled periodically with poor health throughout my life. That way weakness would be familiar and expected. Having always been accustomed to generally good health the contrast between that and how I felt now, came as quite a shock.

From the beginning one of hardest things had been not feeling normal. We couldn't go out to eat with friends, and going to a movie or doing anything half way normal took extreme effort and planning. We had to cancel our weekly Bible Study even though we loved it and we didn't even have to go anywhere because they met at our house. But even that was too hard. So when visitors came to the hospital it helped to make me feel slightly more normal.

The hospital had a TV channel that played peaceful music while showing beautiful, serene sights from nature; rivers, forests, mountains, flowers, and oceans. Periodically I looked up and caught one of these scenes and almost gasped from the magnificent beauty on display all over the earth. God who created all this beauty for us to enjoy is a master artist! Contemplating those serene images was a soothing distraction from being stuck in the hospital. More than once I was almost moved to tears by the loveliness of it all. It's physically difficult to be in the hospital but it's also mentally difficult so you have to work hard at finding beauty wherever you can.

I hated having cancer. I hated every single thing about it. But there was one positive aspect and that was the kindness I received from friends and family. I couldn't believe that people actually came to see me in the hospital. You have probably observed by now that I think it is a long, miserable drive to D.C., so I was surprised by everyone who made the effort. Whether it was a visit, a card, a gift card to a grocery store, a check to help with expenses, or prayers, it all meant so much to me.

While I was experiencing the worst possible health problems, I was also experiencing the best of human kindness, often from unexpected sources. It surprised me that some people who knew me well did not take an active interest in what was happening to me. Maybe they didn't know what to say so they didn't say anything, but if not now, when? I had been weeks away from death by starvation, and they very likely might not have had a chance to say something later.

If you ever find yourself in the position of feeling awkward and not knowing what to say to a sick person, I suggest that you don't avoid them. I recommend you just call the person and tell them that you are sorry to hear about what happened to them and you hope they get better. If you are a praying person, tell them you'll pray for them. That's all you need to say. They know you can't do anything about it, and they don't expect you to utter wise words that make everything alright again. But it is still helpful to know that you care enough to say something even if it's only that you are sorry to hear about it and hope they get better. It may also be your last opportunity to mend broken relationships and improve the peace of mind of the patient as well as yourself. You may live to regret it if you don't say something while you still have the opportunity. But it was equally surprising when people who did not really know me, actively helped me in one way or another, and that happened much more frequently than I ever would have predicted.

When they finally started feeding me broth and liquid my rerouted plumbing gurgled and sputtered in a very uncomfortable manner, but at least it was working. They were intravenously giving me so much fluid that my legs became swollen and too heavy for me to lift to get in and out of bed without Morris's help. But things were starting to work more or less the way they were supposed to so finally on September 19th I was released from the hospital. That was a happy day! My plentiful cancer had not been diminished one bit, but at least I could eat now, and starvation wasn't an immediate concern.

Morris was always trying to think of ways to lift my spirits and do something enjoyable so on the way home we stopped at the Sweet Frog frozen yogurt shop in Leesburg. It was about all I could do to stand upright and walk the short distance into the shop. On the way in, my coworker, Laurie, who was on her lunch break saw us and came by to ask how I was doing. The odds are against running into her at that exact place and time; it goes beyond coincidence and shows me that God is interested and involved in my life. She was happy to see that I was out of the hospital and said she would pass on the good news at work.

HOME, SWEET HOME !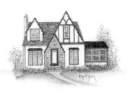

It felt so great to be home, but I was also extremely weak and walking was harder than ever. Morris opened the front door to our house and suggested I head up to bed which sounded good to me. He had to make a quick trip to the post office so I started to go upstairs by myself. I might as well have been climbing Mount Everest! I stopped halfway up and wondered if this had been a bad idea. The potential existed for collapsing; falling down the stairs and tearing open my incision. I had never been so weak in my entire life! It was an unpleasant sensation but one that would continue to be the 'new normal' in the coming months. I finally successfully made it up the stairs and into bed. Being at home and sleeping in my own bed was heavenly! The pain and discomfort caused by that surgery made having babies seem to me like no big deal in comparison.

The next day, Morris took me out for lunch at Magnolia's, a moderately upscale local restaurant that we went to sometimes on special occasions. He wanted to celebrate our escape from the hospital and do something entertaining to take my mind off of being a cancer patient. I learned much later that because my surgery turned out so badly, Morris expected that I wasn't going to live much longer so he wanted to do nice things with me and for me for as long as he could. I don't blame him; at that point it did not look likely that I would recover. At least I would never have bet money on it.

We were both deprived of sleep in the hospital. With all the constant noise and interruptions, it's hard to sleep or even rest. So we slept a lot the next few days, catching up. Strangely, eating was exhausting to me. Things had been so rearranged inside me that it must have taken a lot of energy for my body to figure out how to process food, because as soon as I ate I always needed a nap.

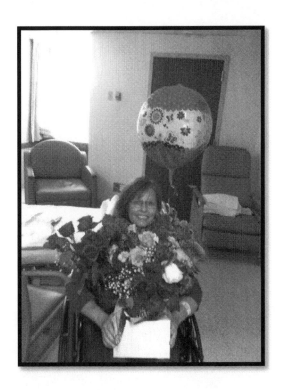

Escaping from the Hospital

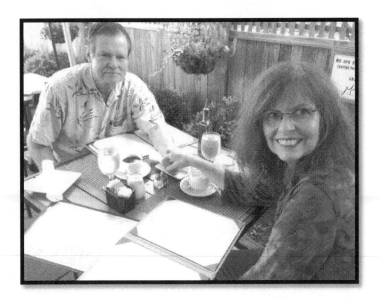

Celebrating escape from the hospital at Magnolia's

If I just sat at a table or on the couch I felt fairly normal, but once I start walking around I felt weak and shaky. The next night we went to a local Greek deli for dinner. I sat down at a table while Morris ordered. The owner asked Morris 'what's wrong with your wife? Is she on drugs?' Who says things like that?! I was mortified! I was trying so hard to look and act 'normal' but I was anything but normal just then. At that time about all I could manage was to eat and then sleep.

But I still felt like I was surrounded by angels. My friend, Missy, had flowers sent to our house several times. My friend, Lesley, came by to get me caught up on the latest news at work.

When we still lived in California our good friends Paul, Barbara and their children, Joleen, and, Justin, lived in our neighborhood, only a couple of blocks away. Our son, Paul, frequently played with their son, Justin, and for a couple years Morris and I played pinochle every weekend with Paul & Barbara. We've been family friends since the early 1980's and by coincidence shortly after we moved to Virginia, they moved to Camp Hill, Pennsylvania, about two hours away.

When they heard I was too sick to do any housekeeping, they drove down to clean our house. They didn't ask us whether we would like them to do it, they told us they were going to do it. On the one hand I couldn't imagine anything kinder or more urgently needed! On the other hand, it was a very humbling experience. It's not easy to let someone else clean up your mess and not feel embarrassed that it got so out of hand. But they didn't seem to be shocked, or if they were they didn't rub it in.

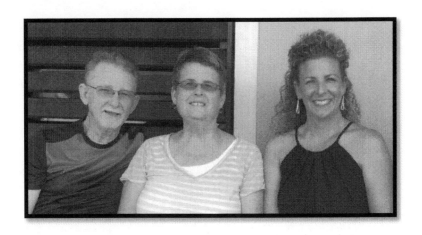

Longtime family friends, Paul, Barbara & Joleen

The three of them spent 10 hours cleaning our house!!! They cleaned the yucky shower and the fridge and scrubbed the kitchen floor on their hands and knees. It was hard for me to sit there like a bump on a log while they worked so hard, but I soon understood that they wanted to do it, and my messy house did not seem to disturb them nearly as much as it did me. It felt so good to have a clean house, and their thoughtfulness was unforgettable!

I worked in a botanical garden in California for 4 years where my primary responsibility was caring for flowers. I love flowers so I was disappointed to be unable to work in the yard or plant seasonal flowers. Paul and Joleen came again a couple weeks later, this time to do some much needed seasonal yard work (pruning, hedging, raking, etc.) and they brought along some mums to add a bit of seasonal fall color, which was a big deal to me.

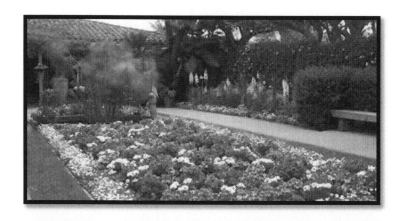

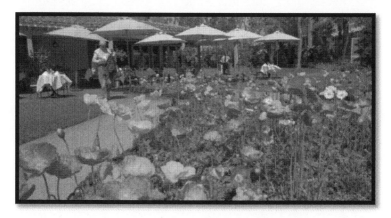

Sherman Gardens, my dream job where my job
was caring for seasonal flowers like these
Martha Washington Geraniums and Iceland Poppies.

Morris was not just sitting around while these other things needed to be done; on the contrary he was doing all his normal tasks as well as mine, along with caring for an invalid. In Morris' father's last days, Morris and I took care of him and that was our first experience as caregivers. It was surprising how there constantly seemed to be something that needed to be done.

Fortunately, Morris was able to work from home which was a blessing since he was also a full time caregiver. He took care of mowing and yard work, but there is extra pruning and trimming that needs to be done a couple times a year and I always did that. It wasn't Morris' normal task and he wasn't familiar with it. Being a caregiver is much more work than might be expected and interruptions make it hard to get much else done.

As a side note, if you know someone who has cancer and you would genuinely like to help, the best approach would be to decide what you are actually willing to do (yard work, laundry, vacuuming, take out the trash, meals or whatever you are comfortable with). Then ask the patient when you can come over to do it. When you have cancer there are many things you want to attend to but you are simply unable to do it.

Friends offer to help and you know they are sincere, but it's hard for the patient to ask, "Hey, could you come over and vacuum now?" That's probably never going to happen so it would be better if you gently force yourself upon them, like Paul, Barbara and Joleen did. Your help is most likely urgently needed, and even strongly desired but it's really hard to ask for help. It just feels like too much of an imposition.

DR. TUAN

Dr. Tuan was now part of our treatment team. Morris and I both felt really good about him and wanted his participation in deciding what our next steps should be. He was the one doctor that we actually enjoyed talking to. He spent a significant amount of time with us, much longer than we had come to expect from other doctor visits.

He helped us think things through (the positives and negatives of all the alternatives). He said that if I opted for chemo he would be able to support me in that and help to minimize the side effects. If I chose not to do chemo he could support me in that as well. I guess that would mean helping me be less uncomfortable in the process of dying.

While we were in the waiting room of Dr. Tuan's office a young woman had just finished her appointment and entered the waiting room. She was young, maybe in her 30's or 40's, far too thin, with a pale complexion and sunken eyes. She wore a cap to cover her hairless head, and her stomach protruded because she had ascites. Our eyes met briefly and she quickly averted her eyes, obviously self-conscious about her appearance. I was so sorry that I made her feel uncomfortable because I strongly identified with her. My condition wasn't much better than hers. I felt as if we were both in the same place. I had so much empathy and understanding for her but was unable to express it.

Dr. Tuan was very kind and compassionate. As gently and tactfully as possible, he said that we'll all die sometime and the important thing was quality of life until then. Basically, in a kind way he was saying that I was fighting an impossible battle and I should not make myself suffer through uncomfortable treatments that wouldn't help me anyway. Better to try to be as comfortable as possible for as long as possible until the end came.

Part of the problem with electing to do chemo was that even if I chose that option my body might not be able to handle it. Sometimes people do not make it through chemo even though they had planned to. So there was good reason for his advice. Dr. Tuan said that most of his patients who chose chemo did not suffer the same debilitating side effects of chemo that others did, and they didn't require a lot of additional medications because of Dr. Tuan's treatment.

A week after I got out of the hospital we went back to D.C. to talk to my surgeon. He seemed pleased with how the surgery turned out. My appetite had improved, and ascites had decreased (in fact they never returned after that point) and that was a very big deal. Dr. Steves recommended that I follow up with chemo. He also suggested that if I did chemo there was a possibility of attempting another surgery in 6 months or so to try again to remove more cancer. The prospect of another surgery was almost too horrible to contemplate just then. Surgery and chemo are both hard and I could go through this painful process and still not get better as Dr. Tuan had cautioned.

I really needed to gain weight and Morris was frequently offering me pies and desserts, trying to fatten me up. He asked me if there was anything at all that I felt like eating because my taste buds had still not readjusted to normal food yet. I said, "Maybe Lemon Meringue Pie". So as Morris made his first Lemon Meringue Pie, I sat in the kitchen telling him what to do. I didn't know it at the time, but he was altering the recipe! More lemons, less water for one thing. Messing with recipes can yield unhappy results, but Morris's Lemon Meringue Pie is the best I've ever had!

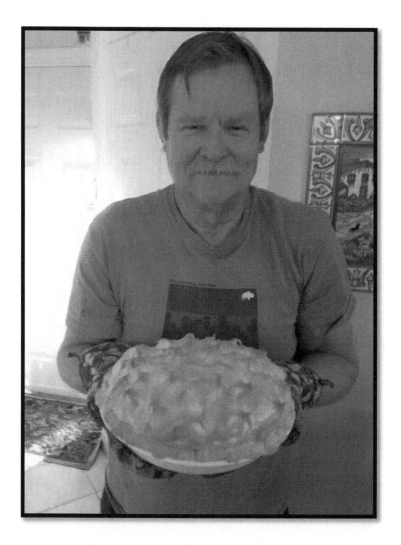

Morris' famous Lemon Meringue Pie!

As a side note, sometime after I recovered from cancer I compiled a cookbook filled with all the best recipes I have accumulated over a lifetime, "Recipes for Most Normal People or Carol's Coveted Collection," (available on Amazon by searching for the title or my name). Morris' Famous Lemon Meringue Pie is one of the best recipes in the book!

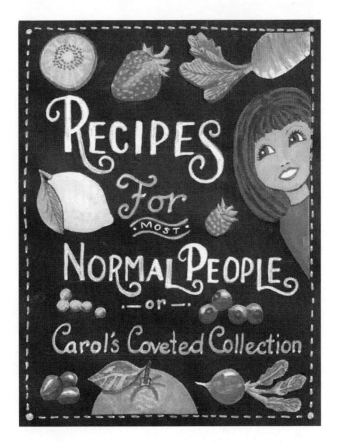

The cover I drew for my cookbook
(I use it daily; it's the best, even if I do say so myself! ☺)

Vicki, from Purcellville Baptist Church set us up with a page on the takethemameal.com website, but it is not limited to people who attend PBC, anyone could use the site. They encouraged me to pass the information along to anyone else who might like to bring us a meal. I didn't even know many of the people who signed up. As I've said before, one thing you find out having cancer is that people are a whole lot more kind and giving than you would ever have imagined. My friends were so kind and supportive, but even people I didn't know were willing to help me out!

As expected, my oncologist recommended chemo and we finally decided to try it, but I still needed a little more time to recover from my first major surgery. Chemo is very rough on the body. The veins get worn and collapse if exposed to it too many times which is why they installed a chemo port under the skin in my upper chest. A tube threaded through my juggler vein and emptied into my heart. That way as the chemo dripped into the heart it was immediately flushed out into the bloodstream where it was diluted more quickly and a little less damaging. Doesn't that sound creepy? It sounded very creepy to me because now I was going to have a chemo port!

To install a chemo port they made a 1" incision in my chest and a 1/2" incision in my neck and ran a 7" piece of plastic tubing down to my heart. Sounded dreadful but it was painless. Unfortunately, it was not painless after the anesthesia wore off. It was completely buried under my skin, so if it weren't for the scar you might never know it was there. When they needed to give me chemo, draw blood or even set me up for a CAT scan, they just poked a needle through my skin into the port and that's it. It made it a little easier for the nurses, but also easier for me. Having been poked countless times in the hospital and being left swollen and black and blue in multiple places I thought this was a good idea even though I wished I didn't need to have it.

Dr. Rajendra said he would be using a combination of Carboplatin and Taxol, administered weekly. Getting a smaller, weekly dose was easier on the body although it was more time consuming to go weekly. Dr. Rajendra said it would take 4-8 weeks to tell what my hair loss might be like. It might just thin a little and I might not need a wig. After he walked out of hearing range the nurse said, "Get a wig."

Nausea and vomiting almost always accompanies chemo and he had medications that could alleviate that. We asked if he would be willing to work with Dr. Tuan, my acupuncturist doctor to control side effects, and he said that he could work with that.

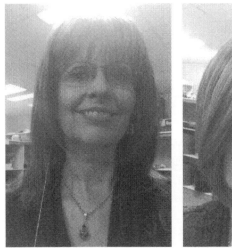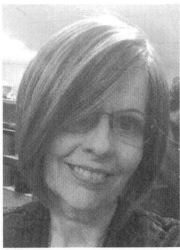

Before getting chemo we picked up a couple wigs at a wig shop. It wasn't certain at that point whether or not I'd lose my hair, but I did, and it happened fairly quickly.

A nurse talked us through what to expect from chemo. It was sort of disheartening that I finally was resorting to chemo. I never wanted to for all the reasons that the nurse explained in the briefing. Taxol sometimes caused allergic reactions so they wanted me to take 3 anti-allergy medications the first couple of times to make sure nothing happened. It can also cause neuropathy (nerve damage in the extremities, painful tingling in the fingers, etc.) If I started to have trouble buttoning a blouse I was to let them know. They did not warn me that chemo would disrupt my sleep, but soon that became a major problem. They wanted to give me 40 minutes' worth of meds before chemo that were supposed to help me cope with the negative side effects, then 1 ½ hours of Taxol, 1 ½ hours of Carboplatin every Friday.

Chemo messes up all your blood counts, there are fewer white blood cells which suppresses the immune system. The count of red cells is lower making you anemic, oxygen deprived and fatigued. Platelets might also be lower making you prone to bleeding and bruising. I could get diarrhea, and nausea and vomiting is very common. If I got a fever of more than 100.5 F or any other unusual symptoms I was to call them. It was difficult for me to see how something that caused this much damage was supposed to help me get better.

The only reason I was willing to take chemo was because there appeared to be no other alternative at this point. My lab work showed that I was anemic, which meant my red blood counts were low. Red blood cells carry oxygen so that explained why I was so tired and out of breath; my body wasn't getting enough oxygen. Just walking to the restroom left me gasping for air! Cancer is one of the things that can cause anemia, and my recent surgery could have also contributed to it. The walls of the small intestine absorb water and the digested nutrients into the bloodstream and now I had a lot less intestines to absorb the nutrients needed to produce red blood cells. The surgeon had removed 60% of my large intestines and 40% of my small intestines.

Chemo was likely to make my anemia worse because chemo targets the cells that divide rapidly (cancer cells) but it also goes for the bone marrow because those cells also divide rapidly. Blood cells are produced in the bone marrow so you end up with fewer white blood cells and a compromised immune system, fewer red blood cells which causes anemia and fewer platelets which creates tendency to bleed or bruise easily. Chemo is poison that is supposed to be selective in what it kills (mainly cancer) but it's not all that selective and it does a whole lot of collateral damage. That is exactly what I expected, and that is why I tried so hard to avoid chemo.

CHAPTER 4

THE HEALING POISON

My oncologist had me take some medications the night before I started chemo to prevent nausea, vomiting and a possible allergic reaction to chemo. One of them was a steroid, one was Benadryl and the other Zantac. In the morning, about the time we were walking into the doctor's office it struck me that I felt surprisingly good for a change. I was usually ready for a long nap right after breakfast (not kidding) but that day I felt alert and energetic. I had been having trouble sleeping for a couple weeks but the night before chemo I slept like a log. We mentioned these things to the nurse and she said the extra energy might be the result of the steroids and the sleep the result of the Benadryl.

The doctor's office has 10 seats for administering chemo, and each person is allowed to have one visitor. The nurse put a needle into the port that was installed the previous week and from then on it was pretty simple. Through an IV she first ran some more of the same meds they gave me the night before, then Taxol and Carboplatin, the two types of chemo. The whole process took about 4 hours, but they take it more slowly the first time. It was no big deal, I felt comfortable the entire time. However I would not feel the effects of it for a day or two. The night after my first chemo I did not sleep at all, in fact I did not sleep even one minute. That was the first time, and the worst time chemo kept me awake, but it would become a recurrent problem.

I hate being nauseous just about more than anything else on the planet, so I really hoped that would be controlled one way or the other. Some people have chemo and suffer debilitating side effects so we would have to wait and see how I would react.

Though I was usually healthy, by now my body had been under attack by cancer for a long time, so I hoped it was still up for the fight. My personal belief is that as long as God has work for me to do, and people for me to bless He will keep me here. If I've done all that I was supposed to do then it's time to go home and that is good too. There are many people I care about and I hated the thought of leaving them behind. So I would continue to make every effort to get well, and leave the outcome to God.

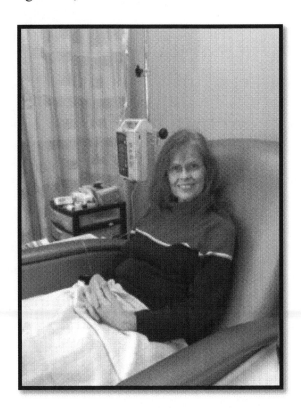

Getting chemo

The Bible records many healing miracles that Jesus performed and it has always interested me that he never used the same technique twice. People have speculated that he kept changing things up because he did not want people to put him in a box and come up with 'magic' formulas for the way things always have to be done. He can do what He wants, how He wants, when He wants and He always does what is best. "For I know the plans I have for you, says the Lord. They are plans for good and not for disaster, to give you a future and a hope."[6]

Jesus healed one blind man by spitting into the dirt and making mud and then putting the mud on the man's eyes and praying. My friend, Kathy, pointed out to me that the blind man probably would have preferred a different, less bizarre and messy method for restoring his sight, but he got his sight back, which was the objective. I had been so vehemently opposed to chemo for such a long time and only decided to go with it when I ran out of options. Now I was forced to adjust my attitude. God is the Sovereign King of the Universe. If He chose to use chemo to heal me He could. And so I waited to see if that was what He was going to do.

My employer, the Town of Leesburg, generously allows employees to share their sick leave with coworkers who need it under certain circumstances, and the Town allowed my coworkers to donate some of their sick leave to me. I had saved quite a bit of sick and vacation leave but by that time it was nearly gone. I didn't really know exactly how much leave my friends gave me, but from what my friend, Lesley, told me it was substantial. Lesley gave me a week of leave herself! When Lesley told me about their

---

[6] Jeremiah 29:11 (NLT)

generosity, it was so unexpected that I began to cry and Morris rushed out of his office to find out what was going on. Eventually I learned that my coworkers contributed enough of their leave to allow me to receive full pay and benefits for six months!

That seemed almost too good to be true. I will forever hold the Town of Leesburg in the highest regard because they have intentionally and compassionately set in place policies that really do have the best interest of the employees in mind.

I had trouble falling asleep that night, but not for the usual reasons. I comfortably lay in bed smiling and thinking of and praying for the good people I worked with until 1:00 AM. But it was pleasant, even enjoyable. Having people mad at you can keep a person awake from stress, but evidently having friends who are so incredibly kind can keep you awake for joy.

Now I was coming up on my 3rd chemo session. I read that one could expect hair loss after 2-3 weeks of chemo so that would be now, but so far I hadn't lost hair. I was still very emaciated and would have been glad to weigh 140 pounds or more again (I never thought I would wish that). I was trying to eat a lot but I still couldn't gain any weight. Chemo was also disrupting my sleep quite a bit, and some nights I hardly slept at all. That was very unusual for me because all my life I have fallen asleep almost as soon as I lay down.

Chemo caused my red blood counts to be very low. That caused my heart to pump rapidly at the slightest exertion as it moved as much oxygen as quickly as possible with the few red blood cells that were available. I felt fairly well if I just sat still on the couch, but the smallest task or effort, like walking to the bathroom had me huffing and puffing, and my heart pounding as if I had been out for a run.

That was disheartening because I like to be active. There were things I would like to do, and I know how to do them, but my frail body wouldn't allow it. I was already tired but it was going to get progressively worse as I had more chemo.

Morris was already doing so much that I didn't want to add to his load by asking him to do more than he was already doing. We had never had professionals clean our house before; it would be nice, but it's expensive! But thanks to the non-profit, Cleaning for a Reason, two maids came for an hour and a half to clean our house once a month for four months while I was having chemo, at no cost to us! If you know anyone having chemo please tell them about this wonderful free service for cancer patients![7] As soon as they verify that the patient is receiving chemo a cleaning can be scheduled. It was such a psychological boost just knowing the house was clean.

By the time I had my 4th chemo session, my hair began to fall out in clumps. I couldn't quite bring myself to completely shave it, but I did have it cut very short. The hairdresser I got was young, and it's likely she had never cut the hair of a chemo patient before. I told her my hair was thinning because of chemo and I wanted it cut very short. She said, "Oh, no! We don't need to do that, we'll just layer it and that will make it look fuller." She ran a brush through my hair and came up with a big handful of hair in her hand. Then she said, "Oh! I didn't know it would do that!" So she cut my hair very short and then I was very glad we had purchased the wigs!

---

[7] HTTPS://CLEANINGFORAREASON.ORG/

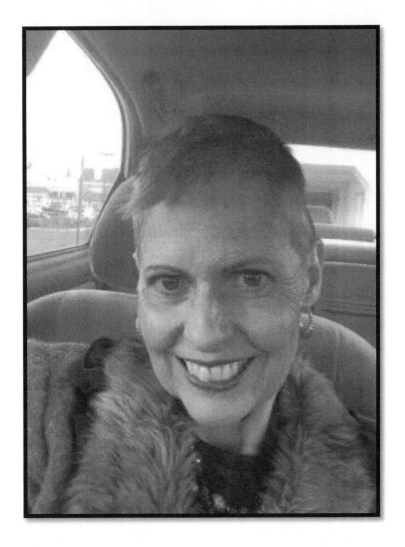

My very short haircut when my hair began to fall out

Chemo is a complete anti-beauty treatment. You not only lose your hair, (all over your body), but your skin becomes very dry, even wrinkled. So the American Cancer Society offers a free class called "Look Good, Feel Better" for women going through cancer treatments. A licensed Cosmetologist teaches how to apply makeup, which I figured I already knew how to do, but they also give each woman $200 worth of free cosmetics and a free, pre-owned wig. So I went to the class, mainly for the freebies and it was well worth it! I also won a $10 gift card to Olive Garden!

Listening to that group of women talk I heard how steroids kept them awake all night, and how tired they were after chemo. They had all lost their hair. The doctors do not really prepare you for all these side effects so it was interesting to know that these problems were not unique to me!

One of the women was a young mother, in her early 20's I'd guess. She had breast cancer and a double mastectomy with reconstructive surgery. It surprised me that someone so young would struggle with this. Another woman was closer to my age. She told us, with tears in her eyes, that when she lost all her hair her daughter said she was going to shave her hair off in a show of solidarity. The mother said, "No, you don't need to actually do that, just saying that you would do it is enough." But her daughter actually shaved her hair off.

At my 6th chemo treatment I also received the results of the previous week's blood test, which was very encouraging. There is a tumor marker for ovarian cancer; the test is called CA 125. A healthy person should have a reading of 35 or less. My very first reading when diagnosed was over 5,000 so not good at all! Months later, before starting chemo, that number had doubled to 10,894. It was definitely going the wrong direction. The results from the test after my 6th chemo session came back 3870, so it had dropped by approximately two thirds! That was still much more than 35, but at least it was going the right direction.

In addition, I had a couple of large, hard lumps (tumors) where there aren't supposed to be any lumps. I noticed a couple of weeks before that they were getting soft and spongy. But by this time, I couldn't feel the lumps anymore; they were gone! So it appeared that the chemo was working and it hadn't been too miserable so far. I lost my hair, was very tired most of the time, and had trouble sleeping, but I never got nauseous. Prayer, Dr. Tuan's herbs and acupressure, and five months of the Gerson Therapy all played a part in that.

As part of my first surgery the surgeon left two clear plastic tubes protruding from my abdomen to drain any ascites if they continued to build up. A week after the surgery he removed one of the tubes by cutting a stitch and pulling it out since very little fluid was draining but he left the other one in just in case the ascites returned.

Prior to surgery I had to go to the hospital 13 times as an out-patient to have ascites drained so having a tube to continuously drain it would have made life a little easier and less painful. But it was also uncomfortable to have a plastic tube protrude from your abdomen for months and always have to watch out that it didn't snag on something. But after the first surgery the ascites never returned, so the doctors agreed it could be removed. It had been there for so long by that time that it would be painful to remove it so I had to go to MedStar in DC and have anesthesia in an operating room. It was a little unpleasant, like a mini-surgery, but at least it was an out-patient procedure and I was glad to get rid of the tube.

By December 15 I was concerned that I might have to have a blood transfusion because the chemo caused my blood counts to drop dangerously low. The nurse said 'they were doing a little happy dance' that morning when my lab results came in because the counts had come up enough that I did not require a transfusion.

But the best news was the results of the CA125 test, the indicator of how much ovarian cancer there was. The healthy range is 0 and 35; I started chemo with my CA125 at nearly 11,000, and now it was down to 227! That was the closest I had been to 35 for a very long time and it was good news indeed! So the cancer was diminishing.

Having cancer is a lot like a wild roller coaster ride; there are many steep ups and downs with some pretty sharp twists and turns in between. You never know what to expect next or if the ride will have a good ending. But the test results were improving and we were cautiously optimistic.

I had made it to a New Year, 2015, which was a milestone because at the beginning in September 2014 I was not at all sure I would live to see November! Now my oncologist, Dr. Rajendra, said I was in the top 10% of responders to this type of chemo! Dr. Rajendra said about 20% of the time women have long term recoveries from ovarian cancer which was good to hear. He recommended that I should go back for a second surgery when chemo was finished. Another surgery was an unpleasant prospect but an expected one. A few months before I had wondered if I would make it to Christmas, but now it looked like I might still celebrate a number of Christmases!

My next CA125 came back at 35! Thirty-five was within the range for a healthy woman! I am the last person on earth who would have recommended chemo, so I was about as surprised by these results as I could possibly be!

Ever since I had surgery I hadn't had any energy and about all I could manage to do was sit on the couch all day with my laptop. A little before Christmas I was getting stronger and was even able to prepare meals and clean up afterwards which would have been utterly impossible a few months earlier. That was about all I could do but it was still progress.

Chemo lowered my white blood cell count to dangerously low levels and since white blood cells are the body's defense to attack germs and viruses, low counts made me susceptible to illness. In fact I could end up hospitalized because my body had so little defense and I was already weak. Because of the low blood count Dr. Rajendra decided to skip my usual chemo until my next blood test, and possibly order a blood transfusion. We seldom went anywhere except to the doctor's office, for fear of exposure to germs. Morris even got me to wear those protective masks when I was out in public. It felt weird but it was better to be safe. My next lab work was better and happily I didn't need the transfusion.

I was almost finished with chemo and had only two sessions left when I learned that my mother, who was 90 years old at the time, had fallen in her bathroom one morning while getting ready for the day. We had recently arranged to have someone come to her home to assist her with shopping, cleaning, and errands but she did not answer the door when her helper came so he notified security. They found her lying on the bathroom floor and it was uncertain how long she had been there, but she was dehydrated. She had to be hospitalized for a few days, but would never be able to live on her own again; she would need to be in assisted living. It was very hard not being able to help her, but at least my sister, Lisa, lived nearby her and could help.

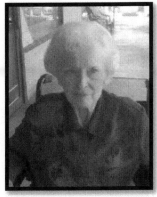

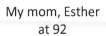
My mom, Esther
at 92

The CA125 results at my next appointment were 20, well within the normal range of 0-35! In February I had the last of 18 chemo sessions which was a huge relief! When I finished chemo we took a quick trip to California to visit family and friends and it was refreshing to do something normal for a change. Fighting a life-threatening illness can be a lonely business, centered on doctor visits (and as I said at the beginning of this book, doctor visits are one of my least favorite things!).

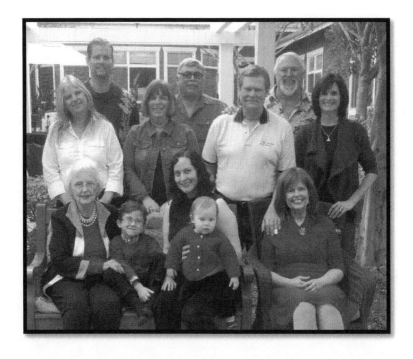

Visiting family in a break between chemo and surgery; front to back, right to left; my mom, grandchildren, Carl and Ruby, daughter-in-law Catherine, me, my sister, Lisa, Marsha (Ken's wife), Morris, Linda (Tim's wife), our son, Paul, and my cousins Ken and Tim

After a brief rest to recover from chemo, my oncologist wanted me to have surgery to remove any remaining cancer while the chemo was still having an effect. He wanted me to schedule surgery 2 to 4 weeks from my last chemo. I was hoping there would be a longer break before surgery because I knew that after I had surgery I would be sitting around recovering again. But the doctor said I had a "Fabulous response" to the chemo, which was encouraging. So I tried not to think about surgery until I had to. I was glad to be done with chemo, and I was glad that for at least a little while I could pretend that I was not a cancer patient, just a regular person.

After a long, cold winter filled with chemo and long weeks with only enough energy to be a couch potato, it felt great to be in Sunny California with temperatures in the 70's. We were able to see my mom's new assisted living home and I hung up all her photos, trying to make her room as cozy as possible. Two months earlier she had been driving and living independently and now she was in assisted living but at least she was being well cared for in a pretty place. We also visited old friends and enjoyed normal activities that are easy to take for granted, until you aren't able to do them.

When we got home our next doctor appointment was with Dr. Steves to discuss my second surgery. February 13 was my last chemo and since then I had gradually felt better and better. In fact I felt so much better that I had been lulled into thinking the cancer had been beaten and that I would just continue to improve. The surgeon agreed there was 'improvement' but said 'that you can't have chemo forever and without the surgery the cancer will come 'roaring back.'

He wanted to operate on March 31. The second surgery would include at least a hysterectomy, and hopefully he would be able to reverse the dreadful colostomy that required constant care. It was horrid and sometimes made me feel like a monster. The doctor wasn't certain he could reverse it, he would have to wait and see, but he hoped to. I really wanted to get rid of that thing and would have been willing to have the surgery just to reverse the colostomy. He would also look for any residual cancer and remove any that he found.

That colostomy probably had saved my life but it was a ghastly thing to live with. Up to 5 times a night I'd wake up abruptly when my hand brushed against the bag and sensed it was full. I would suddenly be wide awake and leap out of bed supporting the full bag for fear it would detach which would have created a horrific mess.

Fortunately that never happened but jumping out of bed 5 times a night was very disrupting to my sleep which was already erratic because of chemo. It was uncomfortable and messy. There were accessories designed to make a good seal around the stoma but they were not always a perfect seal, and would leak and burn the skin. It was very difficult to care for and I could never, ever take a break from it. It was hard enough to take care of it at age 60 and I wondered if I could manage it at all at age 70 or 80.

So the thought that the colostomy could be reversed was something to look forward to, even though I knew what to expect from surgery this time and it would be hard. I left Dr. Steves' office feeling much more subdued. I still had cancer, and it was still life threatening even if for the moment I felt nearly normal.

Dr. Rajendra agreed that surgery was a good idea and that removing as much of the remaining cancer as possible would be wise. He thought it might be advisable to have a little more chemo afterwards, depending on how much cancer remained, but we wouldn't know that until after the surgery. From here on it would be a voyage into the unknown because people vary widely in their response to cancer treatments. About 70% of ovarian cancer patients relapse, and the more advanced the stage, the higher the possibility of relapse. Patients diagnosed at stage IV have a 90 to 95 percent chance of recurrence.[8]

Dr. Rajendra said he has had Stage IV ovarian cancer patients that did really well for a long period of time. But he also has had patients with early stages of cancer that did very poorly. It was impossible to predict how I would respond as time progressed.

Morris was so happy to still have me around that every day was (and still is) like a celebration which has continued to be one of the bright spots. We should all celebrate each new day because none of us knows for sure if we will have another. I guess when you have cancer the odds are so much against you that you become more aware of the reality that time is short and life is fleeting.

Prior to my first surgery I didn't know what to expect so I was fairly unconcerned. This time I knew what was coming and it was a daunting prospect. I wasn't as bothered by the surgery itself, (I would be asleep) as I was by the prospect of being in the hospital for days with bags on my legs, an IV in my arm, and a nasal gastric tube down my throat. The bags were strapped to my legs with Velcro strips and inflated and deflated at random intervals to simulate massage. Their purpose was to avoid blood clots caused by lying in bed for long intervals. It's a

---

[8] HTTPS://OCRAHOPE.ORG/PATIENTS/ABOUT-OVARIAN-CANCER/RECURRENCE/

brilliant invention, but it felt restrictive and I didn't like it. And of course I hated the nasal gastric tube, and the IV inserted in my arm. Last time my arms were both covered with bruises from frequent blood tests. All of it felt very uncomfortable and confining. In any case, I had to have the surgery for more than one reason so I tried to have a positive attitude about it.

Once again I had to have tests prior to the surgery, and once again to spare us the trip to Washington, D.C., Dr. Steves' arranged for his assistant, Belinda, to meet us at Starbucks in Ashburn to pick up my tests. We had only met her one other time, prior to my first surgery but she remembered me and was obviously astonished to see me again. She recalled how advanced my cancer was and like everyone else, she had expected me to have passed on by that time. The first thing she blurted out was, "You look great! I did not expect to ever see you again!" It was blunt and kind of funny, but it was honest.

On March 21, 2015 Morris wished me a "Happy Anniversary!" I had to think a moment and then I realized that on that day one year ago I had been diagnosed with cancer. In March 2014 I wanted to sleep all the time, but on the same day one year later, I took a 3 mile walk. I certainly could never have done that the year before! We still didn't know how this was going to end, and I still had another major surgery coming up in 10 days. But I was alive and doing well, so I did have a Happy Anniversary!

March 31st, 2015 was the date for the second surgery and I was hopeful that this time my recovery would be much faster. The cancer had diminished considerably and would not be as much of a drain on my body's resources. The day before surgery we went over to Purcellville Baptist Church at 1:30 P M for prayer and then headed for our hotel which was nearer to the hospital. We were supposed to be at the hospital at 7:00 AM for 9:00 AM surgery, and were told that the surgery would take around 6 hours more or less. Pastor Kurt and his wife, Shawn, said they would come to DC to pray with us before surgery! That seemed over and above the call of duty to me. It was so early and such a long drive, but it was very much appreciated.

I was allowed to have breakfast the day before the surgery, but for the rest of the day I was only allowed clear liquids and nothing at all after midnight. My most vivid (and painful) memory after my first surgery was an overwhelming desire for water when I first woke up. I asked for ice but was unable to swallow because of three coils of tubing in my mouth (they weren't supposed to be there but we didn't know that at the time). I wasn't able to speak above a whisper for 3 months after due to that terrible tube down my throat. I hoped these types of miserable medical mistakes would not be repeated.

There was a stark contrast between the first and second surgeries. Whereas the first surgery revealed cancer so prolific that it was impossible to distinguish where the cancer left off and my organs began, this time the surgeon was surprised by the complete absence of cancer. He took 18 biopsies but he did not really think that any of it was cancer. He said they were likely just 'shadows.' He wouldn't know for sure until they had been tested, but it was promising news!

This time the nasal gastric tube was inserted correctly, so although I still had a miserable tube down my throat it was not intensely uncomfortable. Last time I awoke from surgery with an overwhelming sense of thirst, but this time we knew to request swabs, small sponges on the ends of sticks so I could moisten my mouth which was all I really needed. These small changes made a huge difference in my in peace of mind and comfort.

Last time large portions of my intestines were removed resulting in an unpleasant colostomy. This time the colostomy was completely reversed so I could use the bathroom like a normal person, which I will never take for granted again! Now I just had to be a good patient so I could be released from the hospital as soon as possible.

The second surgery wasn't nearly as terrible for Morris either. During the first surgery he was required to make a drastic decision to salvage the surgery so that it wouldn't be a complete waste. He recalls it as one of the worst days of his life. This time our friends, Dave, Joe, and Mike and Maria, came to encourage Morris, and Pastor Kurt Bowman and his wife, Shawn came to pray with us before surgery started. Half way through the surgery Dr. Steves sent an optimistic message to Morris to let him know that things were going very well, which made the wait less tense. This time Morris met with Dr. Steves after the surgery in that same little room. Last time Dr. Steves gave him 'bad news and more bad news'. Now he was 'amazed and astonished' at how much everything had changed for the better. He had expected to find some improvement but this was clearly far beyond anything he anticipated.

Dr. Steves kept saying I was a 'Super Star' patient although I didn't feel too much like a super star at the moment. I was attached to tubes, bags, and wires; experiencing numerous hard to define discomforts that individually didn't amount to much but cumulatively were very draining. Dr. Steves was very encouraged though and the good news made the aches and pains a little more tolerable. There really wasn't any sharp pain so since I wasn't using the green button on the self-administered pain medication they discontinued it after a couple of days.

I was so relieved to be rid of the stoma and colostomy, but it would take a very long time for my intestines to readjust. Initially it was as if I had uncontrollable diarrhea, but even after all this time my intestines still have not fully returned to normal, and I'm not certain if they ever will, because more than half of them were removed. But even if that never happens, it's still preferable having a colostomy.

The nurses advised me to walk around in the hospital as much as possible to help get my bowels moving. But I quickly had to stop walking down the hallway because I effectively had no bowel control and could not get to a bathroom fast enough. Wanting to get out of the hospital as quickly as possible, I paced back and forth in my hospital room instead.

Morris told me another piece of news that my surgeon gave him after finishing my surgery. He said it was 'a pleasure to do this surgery.' The previous surgery kept me alive so it wasn't a complete waste, but it didn't remove any of the cancer so in most ways it was a disappointment. But now my condition had improved so dramatically that the surgeon was able to make serious progress which gave him great satisfaction.

Originally my surgeon and oncologist both urged me to have chemo first then surgery, but after getting in there to actually take a look the surgeon said if I had chemo first I would have died. I would have starved before the chemo could have accomplished anything. The doctors had no way of knowing that but God knew it the whole time. All along we had been praying for guidance to make the correct decisions, and God was guiding.

There was one strange new symptom that I woke up with after the second surgery, which had not happened in the previous surgery. Three fingers on my left hand were completely numb. It felt like they were 'asleep' so I shook my hand and opened and closed it, trying to get the blood flowing and the feeling back. Nothing I did had the slightest effect. It was speculated that because I first noticed it immediately after surgery, it might have been caused by being placed in an awkward position for an extended period of time during the lengthy surgery. In any case the numbness did not go away.

This time, thankfully I had a shorter hospital stay, March 31 through April 7. Coincidently, March 31st was the date of my second surgery as well as my last official day of employment by the Town of Leesburg. The Town was a great place to work and I enjoyed all of my coworkers. We had some good times together and I consider them all as personal friends. So it was somewhat sad to be leaving because they had all been incredibly kind and supportive, but we still continue to be friends.

From September 9, 2014, the day I left work to have my first surgery, until March 31, 2015, I had been an employee receiving full pay because of the Town's generous policy of allowing leave sharing, and all the individual employees who generously choose to donate their leave to me. Unforgettable! It was one of many happy and memorable experiences we had in an otherwise dreary year.

They were remodeling the hospital wing that I was in and there were continuous construction noises, but especially at night, and by this time I was the only remaining patient in that wing. So I asked Dr. Steves if he would allow me to go home a day early and much to my delight he said, "Yes!"

I was released from the hospital on April 7th, a beautiful spring day in D.C. The cherry blossoms were in bloom; a fitting symbol of freedom (from the hospital) and new life (without cancer). It wasn't the end of our war on cancer, but a major victory had been won. Against all the odds I was still alive and feeling better all the time.

On April 17, we had a follow-up visit with, Dr. Steves, in Washington D.C. He said that I had 'a marvelous response to the chemo' and was very pleased with how the surgery went. In fact, he told me I was in remission! Remission does not mean the same thing as cured, but it does mean that at least at present there was no detectable cancer. He had no way of knowing if it would stay that way or for how long.

As you know by now, I consider it to be a long, arduous drive to Washington, D.C., so even though there are a lot of things to see there we seldom go. Since we were already there and the Cherry Blossoms were still in bloom, we took the opportunity to park near the Jefferson Memorial to celebrate the beautiful spring day and the excellent news.

The Cherry Blossoms hit their peak the previous Wednesday and it had been raining and windy on the day before which blew away most of the blooms, but there were still plenty of flowers. We walked all the way to the MLK Memorial since we had never seen it before and I estimate we walked 2-3 miles which was the farthest I had been able to walk since having surgery. Things were looking up and we were thankful, and very encouraged!

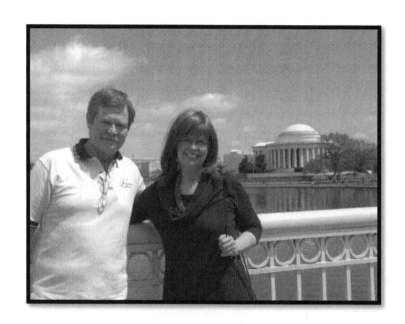

Enjoying the beauty of Spring, and the good news of REMISSION!

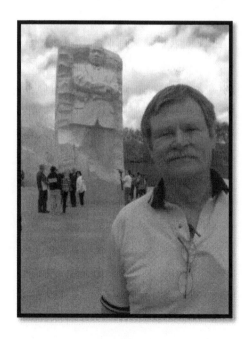

MLK Memorial

Twelve days later I had two more doctor appointments, first with my oncologist, and then my acupuncturist. My surgeon had called me 'a superstar', and now my oncologist was calling me a superstar too. He said my response to chemo was 99.9%; basically it could not have been any better. My acupuncturist said, "To be honest, you have exceeded my expectations." So all three of my doctors were astonished by how well I had done and Morris and I were equally amazed! I don't think I could possibly be that lucky; God healed me, it's a miracle!

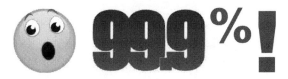

Throughout 2014, I periodically contemplated the surreal and unpleasant possibility that I might not be around in a matter of weeks, or months at the most. That wasn't just because of the diagnosis and the treatments; I sensed that my strength and vitality was rapidly diminishing. Morris didn't say so, but he didn't expect me to last much longer after my first surgery turned out so badly. I cannot overstate what a poor state of health I had been in. But now, astonishingly, I was in remission! It was incredible, unbelievable. A true miracle!

Lots of friends and family were cheering me on and I sincerely appreciated the encouragement, but what I prized even more were their prayers. I believe that prayer is what made the difference, and I thank and credit God with my miraculous recovery. My doctors were clearly blown away; it was obvious that none of them expected me to make it.

They are all highly educated medical professionals with years of experience working with cancer patients. They were all very familiar with what to expect, and none of them expected this outcome! In fact I recently had a routine follow-up appointment with Dr. Rajendra in May 2019. At that time he said, "I can tell you now that when you first came to see me I doubted that you would have more than a few months." And now a few months has turned into a little over 4 years!

Chemo had been very effective so to be on the safe side my oncologist recommended 6 more weekly chemo sessions to knock out any stray cancer cells. He said that about 20% of his ovarian cancer patients go on to live 5 years or more, and he was hopeful that I would be one of them.

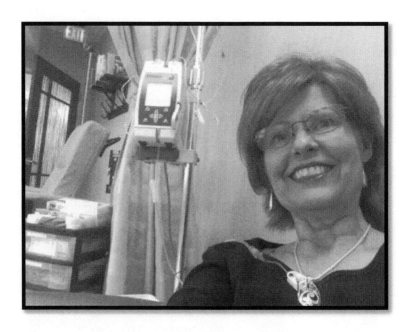

Back to chemo, six more sessions to kill stray cancer cells.

One nasty side effect that often accompanies chemo is neuropathy (nerve damage in the extremities, like fingers and toes that causes them to feel numb or tingly and prickly). Every time I went in for a chemo treatment they asked if I had any neuropathy and up to that point I had always been able to answer, "No". But now all my toes were tingling and it seemed to be getting worse. Chemo was the cause, and there was no guarantee the neuropathy would go away when the chemo treatments were completed.

When I first started working for the Town of Leesburg, my supervisor was John. For 16 years John's wife, Betsy, had been very involved in a cancer society fund raiser called Relay for Life and now she invited us to attend as a cancer survivor and caregiver. It was such a pleasant experience; a huge celebration of life! First they had cancer survivors walk a lap around a track and as they passed between two long columns of well-wishers waving colorful flags, each survivor was announced and how long they had survived.

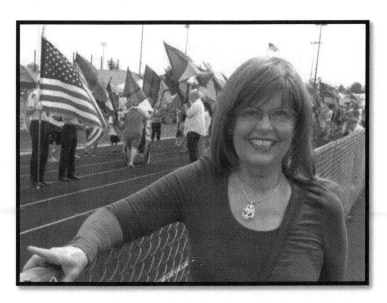

Relay for Life Survivors being acknowledged

Caregivers and survivors were treated to a delicious catered lunch with live music, and a lot of lovely gifts were raffled off. I was amazed that so many people would devote so much time to this worthy fundraiser. It was a beautiful event in every way and I was happy to be alive to participate in it!

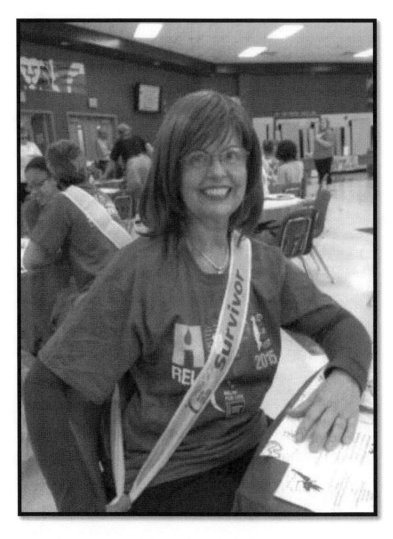

Lunch at the Relay for Life

Cancer, two surgeries and chemo had been very hard on my appearance but now I was beginning to gain weight and I had grown about ¾" of grey hair. It was June which is hot and humid in Virginia so wearing a wig felt like wearing a warm winter hat; stifling! I just couldn't stand it anymore so I stopped wearing the wigs and actually had the nerve to go out in public au natural. Surprisingly nobody looked twice.

I figured if people knew me, then they would also know why my hair looked that way. If they didn't know me then they would just think I had unusual taste in hairstyles and they wouldn't care anyway. And I always had the option of wearing a wig if I wanted to blend in and look more 'normal', but I never wore a wig again after that.

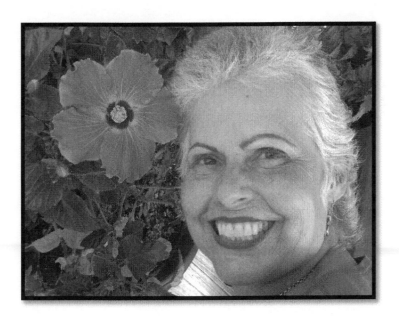

My post-chemo hair

134

I had my last chemo session in June of 2015. My platelet count was too low, which meant I could easily start bleeding and so they did not give me both chemo treatments that last day, only one of them. I was told to monitor myself for bleeding and have another blood test in a few days. Then in a couple weeks when the platelets came back up I could have my chemo port removed (an outpatient surgery).

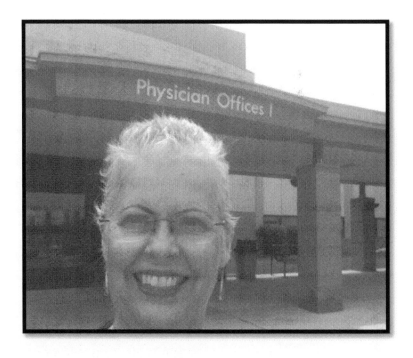

Last chemo! Yay!

CHAPTER 5

A NEW LEASE ON LIFE

From then on my oncologist would just monitor me, no more chemo or surgery! I was very happy and very thankful. Coming that close to dying changed my perspective on a lot of things. Don't sweat the small stuff, and it's all small stuff compared to almost dying. I also learned that when the chips are down, 'stuff' doesn't matter much. People are the important thing!

About a year after this ordeal was all over with my oncologist advised me to take a genetic test to determine if I had the BRCA1 or BRCA2 gene. Seven out of ten women with the BRCA1 gene develop breast cancer. Three out of ten women with the BRCA1 gene develop ovarian cancer. I had the test and it turned out that I have the BRCA1 gene. Very bad news, but at least it explained why I got ovarian cancer, and this information proved helpful to other members of my family, who as it turned out also have the gene.

Years earlier my cousin, Inger, in Norway was diagnosed with breast cancer. Genetic testing revealed that she had the BRCA1 gene, and she wrote to me at that time advising me to be tested. Three other cousins also had the gene. Later I learned that four of my Norwegian aunts died of either breast or ovarian cancer.

The genetic test is very easy to take. It's just a blood test, and in Norway the test is free. The head of the cancer research department at Oslo University Hospital (the largest in Scandinavia) told Inger that they find it useful to study families like ours and that our family history was "very interesting". So they also offered the test for free to my sister, Lisa, and I. We have two additional relatives that tested positive for the BRCA1 gene, 12 in all that I know of (if my father and I are counted, because I couldn't have BRCA1 unless he had it too). So the gene is indeed very strong in our family which is both 'very interesting' and very disturbing.

I don't think I grasped the magnitude of what having the BRCA1 gene meant when Inger told me about it. I just don't think I 'got it.' I was younger, perpetually healthy, and didn't see the need for it at that time. I also had a slight concern that if indeed I did have a genetic predisposition toward some major health problem, perhaps I could be denied insurance coverage as a pre-existing condition. I don't really think that would have been a problem; how would anyone even find out if the test was performed in Norway? Maybe I was just too lazy to take the time and effort to send the test in since I was still young enough to feel invincible.

If I had taken the test for BRCA1 back when Inger first told me about it, it's very unlikely that I would have gotten ovarian cancer. By simply removing the ovaries, which is an out-patient procedure, I could have avoided the entire nightmare! If I understood then what I know now I would have gladly accepted the offer to test for BRCA1, but hind sight is 20/20.

I was increasingly feeling more 'normal' and normal felt great after being continuously fatigued and debilitated for over a year! Be glad if you feel 'normal'! Once the chemo port was out, I started acupuncture to see if something could be done for the neuropathy in my fingers and toes. To begin with Dr. Tuan measured my meridians (the biological circuits that transmit energy throughout the body) with an electronic device to see where the energy flow was off. Then the doctor placed about 8 pins at different locations on my back and left them there for 15 minutes. I rolled over and he placed about 12 more pins, mainly on my arms and feet. It wasn't uncomfortable at all; it could barely be felt. Afterwards he explained the chart of the measurements he took and what the goal was in order to stay healthy and not have a relapse. It made a lot of sense, and it was measurable. It was much different than Western medicine and it was fascinating.

We went for acupuncture treatments every other week, and it really did help. My toes improved by about 50% and so did my fingers. Three fingers on my left hand had all felt completely numb and remained that way well after the surgery, but now they were doing a lot better. Nerves only grow a couple inches a year so they are very slow to heal. After one particular acupuncture session, I went in with three partially numb fingers and came out with only two that were still numb! The one session restored my middle finger completely back to normal! Dr. Tuan said the middle finger was connected to a different nerve then the other two fingers.

By this time I had a whole lot of experience with Western Medicine. Acupuncture is much less invasive than most Western Medicine, and now I know that it really does work! Unfortunately, like most other naturopathic treatments, acupuncture was not covered by my insurance. I don't understand why they don't cover it because it works!

In October of 2013 before I knew that I had cancer, Morris and I hiked to Maryland Heights Overlook for an impressive view of Harpers Ferry, WV, where three states converge; Virginia, West Virginia and Maryland, along with two major rivers; the Shenandoah and Potomac.

At that time I probably had cancer without knowing it yet; I wouldn't find out until five months later. One year later I was recovering from my first major surgery and doing extremely poorly. I could barely even walk to the bathroom. My doctors did not expect me to survive; and to be honest, neither did my husband or I. It looked like I would never ever be able to make that hike again.

But in October 2015 we successfully did take that hike again! We hiked partly just to do something fun on a spectacular fall day, but we also did it to celebrate that I was well enough to do it! Victory!

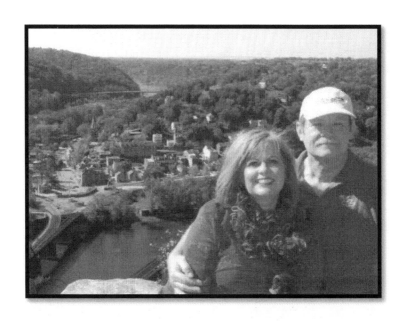

Harpers Ferry, October 2013 Pre-cancer diagnosis

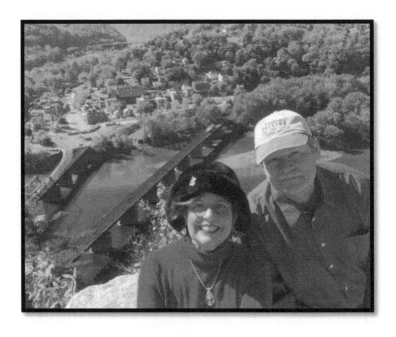

Harpers Ferry, October 2015, Remission!

CHAPTER 6

THE BEST THERAPY

NATUROPATHIC VS. ALLOPATHIC MEDICINE

Please note that I don't have any medical training and I'm not qualified to give medical advice. All I know is my first-hand experience with the cancer treatments I actually used, and the effect they had on me personally. The following comments are only my anecdotal opinions and not medical advice.

I used the Gerson Therapy for the first 5 months after I learned I had cancer. It is a completely natural or naturopathic cancer treatment. Even though it was natural, it was neither simple nor easy; in fact it was so much work that I would never have been able to do it without Morris' help. I would not have even attempted it.

When I began using the Gerson Therapy I experienced immediate and measureable improvement. For one thing I did not feel the need to sleep around the clock. I was able to work at a full time job for another five months, and felt fairly normal again. The severe ascites I had been experiencing also slowed to a near stop, and they did not return for months. My lab work also improved dramatically.

Even though it was not enough to lead to my full recovery, I remain completely convinced that the Gerson Therapy works, for some people at least. Some of the people we met at the Gerson clinic have passed on by this time, while others have returned to vibrant health.

I am especially thinking of our friend, Todd, who had stage IV melanoma when we met. Allopathic medical doctors, who were specialists in melanoma, only gave him a 1% chance for recovery, nearly zero! Melanoma is a particularly aggressive form of cancer and there is almost no hope for recovery from advanced cases, just as Todd was told.

Yet today Todd is completely healthy and active, frequently enjoying his favorite pass-time, scuba diving. If Todd were the only person I knew who experienced this radical recovery, that would be enough to convince me that Gerson has a lot of merit as a cancer treatment, but he is not the only one. You can watch a YouTube of Todd discussing his recovery by searching for "Todd's recovery from stage IV melanoma with Gerson Therapy."[9]

Eventually the Gerson Therapy no longer worked for me because it is a food based therapy and the cancer had permeated my intestines so completely that I could no longer process food. Yet even at that point, at my first visit with my new oncologist, Dr. Rajendra, he repeatedly said, "I have to admit I am very impressed with your labs." He qualified that by saying that the Gerson Therapy might be responsible for my great lab work, but it might also just be my naturally strong constitution; an argument could be made either way.

---

[9] HTTPS://WWW.YOUTUBE.COM/WATCH?V=WOQNV7OREIA

But neither Western Medicine nor Naturopathic Medicine has a 100% success rate. We all know people who sought cancer treatment from medical doctors and recovered, as well as people who did not make it, regardless of what treatment type was used.

One reason it's so hard to find 'the' cure for cancer is because cancer is not just one illness. There are many forms of cancer and each type requires a different treatment regimen. For example, our friend, Tim's, cancer could not be treated by chemo therapy, but mine could. Some cancer patients don't get chemo, but they do get radiation, others just take pills.

At the Gerson Clinic we met a number of people who were there specifically because Western Medicine had already failed them. It either hadn't done enough, or it had worked for a time but they relapsed. Some of those patients did not make it, but others recovered using Naturopathic Medicine after Western Medicine could do no more.

It's easy to find stories like that of Bailey O'Brian who at 20 years of age was told by her oncologist at NYU Hospital that she had seven months to live. At 17 she had been diagnosed with melanoma cancer and she thought she had beaten it, but two years later it was back and even stronger than before. By then it was inoperable, and Western Medicine could no longer help her.

Bailey stated that it was a death sentence, but she and her parents fought on in any way they could, whether or not the FDA or even her own doctors approved. They went to CHIPSA clinic in Tijuana and used a variety of naturopathic treatments, including the Gerson Therapy. As of March, 2019 Bailey has been in remission for 5 years.[2]

Leslie Bocoski was diagnosed with terminal ovarian cancer in 1985 and given less than one year to live. She used the Gerson Therapy and 33 years later she is still telling people about her remarkable recovery against all odds. These are not uncommon stories; they are only a couple of examples. Naturopathic medicine offers many inspiring accounts of people who recovered even after Western Medicine had failed them.[3]

If any type of treatment worked every time for every cancer patient that news would spread like wildfire, and before too long everyone would be exclusively using that treatment. Unfortunately, it's not that simple; cancer is complicated. Not only is each type of cancer different but people are different too.

What might be the perfect treatment regimen for one person might not be as successful on another person. The best therapy is the therapy that will work for you, personally. But finding the treatment that will work best for you seems to require some guesswork. Morris and I are Christians so we prayed about all our medical decisions and we believe God directed us.

After I stopped using the Gerson Therapy, I had surgery (without chemo first) and that appeared to be a complete disaster because the cancer had fused to all my organs and the surgeon couldn't remove any cancer. But he was able to remove the parts of my intestines that were blocked by cancer which saved me from immediate and certain death by starvation. It also stopped the ascites as the surgeon had hoped, and that was very significant.

Later my surgeon admitted that if I had chemo first as they originally recommended, I would have died. I would have starved before chemo had time to do anything. I only point that out because all of my doctors said I should have chemo before the surgery. But now it was clear that if I had chemo before it would have failed. Doctors always make their best recommendations, but they are not always right. In my case I don't believe for a moment that was just a lucky chain of events; God was directing our steps.

Next I had many months of chemo treatments, which happened to be a perfect match for me. This came as a big surprise. Previously I had heard nothing but horror stories about chemo treatments (with the one exception of Shawn). However, on me it worked extremely well. At first my oncologist said I was in the top 10% of responders to that chemo, and later he said I was in the top .01% of responders.

That was outstanding news but please note that it also means that 99.9% of his patients do not respond as well to it as I did. That's why in some ways it seems to me that there is an element of chance or guess work in selecting the right cancer treatment and that not all treatments work equally well on all people. The combinations of chemo that my doctor used just happen to work especially well with BRCA1 cancers.

At my second surgery, no cancer was found and I was told I was in remission. But the surgeon, Dr. Steves, clearly had not expected that; he was very surprised. So that was not 'normal' or 'likely.' In fact it was very unusual and unexpected.

When I began my battle with cancer I was certain that natural methods were far superior and allopathic methods were pretty much no good at all. But hopefully by now you can understand at this point why I don't feel confident recommending one treatment over another. Both naturopathic and allopathic medicine seem to work very well, sometimes, on some people, and neither of them work all of the time on all people.

So about all I am able to suggest is that you find a doctor or a team of doctors that you feel comfortable with and carefully evaluate their recommendations. Perhaps you should also consider a combination of naturopathic and allopathic treatment, like I eventually did having an oncologist and an acupuncturist. I really think that chemo was much easier for me than for most people because of my acupuncturist's treatments, and possibly the 5 months I spent on the Gerson Therapy.

So what is the best therapy? The best therapy is the one that will work for you. If you opt for Western Medicine and it ever gets to the point that it's not working, you might consider switching to Naturopathic Medicine or conversely from Naturopathic to Western.

Basically exhaust all the options and never, ever give up. My experience is that you can never be certain what is going to work best in your case, so if one treatment method stops helping, try something else. I could have given up when Gerson stopped working for me, or when my first surgery had such a grim outcome because the prognosis looked very bleak indeed back then. But then I wouldn't be here anymore. The only time you can be sure that you are not going to recover is when you stop trying to get better. Never, Never, Never Give Up!

NEVER
NEVER
NEVER
GIVE UP

This plaque sat on a shelf in my office while I worked and fought cancer. I often glanced at it and considered its message. Sometimes the situation appeared to be completely hopeless and my sign seemed unbelievable and ridiculous, but we did not give up, and miraculously, I recovered.

CHAPTER 7

GOD AND LIFE

The strength of the vessel can be demonstrated only by the hurricane, and the power of the Gospel can be fully shown only when the Christian is subjected to some fiery trial. If God would make manifest the fact that "He gives songs in the night," He must first make it night.

—William Taylor[10]

By September 2014, my survival appeared highly unlikely. But then to my great surprise, everything changed and I recovered. Nobody is more surprised than I am because I know how weak I was. My recovery is nothing less than a genuine miracle in the Biblical sense. However, other very good people I know did not recover and it is a complete mystery why I got well while those other good people did not.

After my first surgery revealed that the cancer was much too far advanced for the surgeon to do anything other than unblock my intestines, a safe bet would be that I was not going to make it, and I understood that. As mentioned previously, that is when I wrote the following;

10

HTTPS://WWW.CROSSWALK.COM/DEVOTIONALS/DESERT/S
TREAMS-IN-THE-DESERT-JUNE-7TH.HTML

"I would like to say, that we have not given up. Things don't look good. In fact they almost could not look any worse than they do right now. However God has numbered my days before there were any of them. He knows how many hairs are on my head and has counted all my tears and kept them in a bottle. He is all knowing and all powerful. I know I have multitudes of people praying for me, they tell me so all the time. We still intend to look into any other possible life saving man made measures, but above all we are looking to the Great Physician. No one can keep me here if He wants to take me home, but nothing can take me out if He wants to keep me here either!"

When I wrote those words I didn't know if I would live or die, but either way I knew that I would be fine. It's unthinkable to me to confront anything as grim as cancer without my faith in God. It was essential to my recovery. *I do not believe I would still be alive today without God's miraculous intervention, and the hope and peace He gave me.*

My faith in the Christian God of the Bible is what sustained me from beginning to end throughout the entire ordeal. Jesus said, "be sure of this: I am with you always, even to the end of the age"[11] Without the assurance that God was with me and helping me even at the worst possible moments, it would be entirely reasonable and rational to be afraid! There was a lot to be afraid of! Honestly, I don't know how people get through adversity without His help! He carried me through the deep waters of cancer and without His aid, this story would be very different (not in a good way). That's why it would be

---

[11] MATTHEW 28:20 (NLT)

pointless for me to talk about my struggle with cancer without also talking about how God helped me through it.

The Bible is a perpetual best seller; although it is impossible to obtain exact figures, there is little doubt that the Bible is the world's best-selling and most widely distributed book.[12] There are 2.18 billion professed Christians worldwide, which is about 31.6 percent or nearly 1/3 of the world population[13] In the balance of this book I will explain some of the reasons why the Bible is so helpful to me, and what Christians believe and why they believe it. As a stage IV cancer patient with only weeks to live, I was heading straight into 'the valley of the shadow of death' and I knew it. But because of my faith in God I could still be at peace and 'fear no evil.'[14]

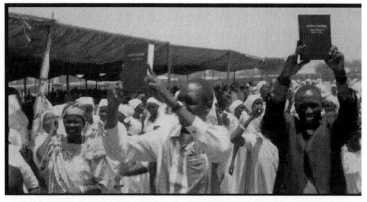

Christians in South Sudan joyfully receiving Bibles

[12]
HTTP://WWW.GUINNESSWORLDRECORDS.COM/WORLD-RECORDS/BEST-SELLING-BOOK-OF-NON-FICTION/
[13] HTTPS://WWW.REFERENCE.COM/WORLD-VIEW/PERCENTAGE-WORLD-CHRISTIAN-4BAEFDA21D3BFCFD

[14] PSALM 23:4 (KJV)

The libraries of the world are filled with books about God, religion and philosophy. All people, in all places, in every century have asked the 'big questions' at various times in their lives. Questions such as; "Why am I here? What is the meaning of life? What is Right and Wrong? What happens after death? Does God exist? Are we just biological machines that make predictable responses to stimuli, or do we have free will and free choice? What is man? What is truth? What is man's responsibility to truth?" They ask these because they are seeking meaning and purpose.

There are an enormous number of books about Christianity for the same reason. All people seek meaning and purpose. The Bible says, "If every one of the things Jesus did were written down, I suppose that even the whole world would not have room for the books that would be written."[15]

From the moment that the nurse informed me that I had stage IV cancer, I understood that my diagnosis was a potential death sentence. But even in that dark moment I was struck by the complete absence of fear. Jesus said, "I am leaving you with a gift—peace of mind and heart. And the peace I give is a gift the world cannot give. So don't be troubled or afraid."[16] I had been caught off-guard by the worst possible news, and without time to think or 'get psyched up,' I was at peace. To me that was extraordinary, and my calm and peaceful response proved to me that my

---

[15] JOHN 21:25 (NLT)
[16] JOHN 14:27 (NLT)

faith is genuine and that I really do believe what I claim to believe.

Even when the cancer progressed to the point that it looked like I was not going to make it, that peace remained. That doesn't mean I was comfortable or happy about it, but I knew that live or die I would be alright. Knowing that my life was in God's hands and I really could not lose either way is what gave me that peace. The members of my immediate family are all Christians, so I would see them again. Leaving them would be hard, but it would not be a permanent condition, and they would also be in God's hands.

Without that hope and assurance there would be nothing to expect but loss; dying would be a disastrous, permanent, hopeless loss. It would be a complete and utter defeat and how could any rational person be at peace about that? The best case scenario would be that death is just the end of consciousness, nonexistence. But even if there is nothing after death, dying could not be understood as anything other than a complete, total and permanent loss of all the good things that were once enjoyed while living.

In my opinion, if there is no God and no life after death, then anything we do in this life is pointless and meaningless. I am not alone in that opinion; it is an opinion shared by many atheistic philosophers. Why live at all? Should we live to have children and perpetuate the human race? Or maybe we should live for pleasure, fun and enjoyment? But life also involves struggles, pain and suffering. If it's all over when we die, what was the point of any of it?

Nihilism is a depressing and hopeless philosophy that declares that nothing has meaning or purpose. It also assumes there is no ultimate higher authority and therefore nothing is morally right or wrong. The Russian author, Dostoevsky, would agree. He wrote "If there is no God - then everything is permitted."[17] If there is no God then there is no standard higher than oneself to say authoritatively that anything is right or wrong. This has caused endless confusion in the modern world. If each person is entirely autonomous and each decides his/her own 'truth' then the variations of 'truth' are infinite and conflict with other people's 'truth' is inevitable.

When everyone invents their own 'truth' it makes it nearly impossible to arrive at a consensus on anything. The best we can hope for is to align ourselves with groups of like-minded people. In that case, what is moral, true and right is not absolute, fixed and certain, but rather is decided by whoever has the largest group and can successfully force their will upon everyone else. And so we end up with 'might makes right.'

In contrast, Christians acknowledge God as the ultimate source of authority, not the State and not fluctuating public opinion. Christians regard the Bible as God's own words and the only infallible source of truth. This is exactly why Communist countries characteristically attempt to suppress Christianity and outlaw Bibles. Christians are commanded in the Bible to be peaceful, law abiding citizens and obey the authorities over them; unless man's laws are unjust and/or conflict with God's laws. In that case they must obey God rather than man. Fortunately for all of us, Christians such as Dr. Martin Luther King Jr. who resisted the South's segregation laws, and the Quakers who helped slaves escape to freedom were willing to suffer imprisonment and persecution rather than obey the unjust laws of man.

---

[17] THE BROTHERS KARAMAZOV, FYODOR DOSTOEVSKY

In 2018, "4,136 Christians were killed for faith-related reasons."[18] That's 344 Christians per month that are killed for their faith globally, although we do not hear much about it in the news. Another source states that 90,000 Christians were killed for their faith in 2016 mainly due to the rise of ISIS![19] Christians are like all other normal people, they want to live peacefully with their family and neighbors, and go about their business. But if there is a conflict between God's laws and man's ideas, they will follow God even at the risk of their lives. That is precisely why oppressive governments view Christians as a threat and strive to prevent them from meeting and having access to Bibles.

LIFE WITHOUT MEANING

More than once I have heard atheist philosophers admit that life without God is a life without meaning. I think anyone who thinks it through logically would have to arrive at that conclusion, and I admire their honesty. One philosopher said; "Man is a useless passion. It is meaningless that we live and it is meaningless that we die."[20] A director/producer said, "The very meaninglessness of life forces a man to create his own meaning."[21] That's because "Man cannot stand a

---

[18] HTTPS://WWW.GATESTONEINSTITUTE.ORG/13813/CHRISTIANS-PERSECUTED-KILLED
[19] HTTPS://WWW.BREITBART.COM/NATIONAL-SECURITY/2017/01/01/REPORT-90000-CHRISTIANS-KILLED-FAITH-2016/
[20] JEAN-PAUL SARTRE
[21] STANLEY KUBRICK

meaningless life."[22] In contrast, "Other men see only a hopeless end, but the Christian rejoices in an endless hope."[23]

Shakespeare can be difficult to understand, it is for me anyway. I had to memorize Hamlet's soliloquy (monologue) in high school which forced me to think about what he was saying. Following are a few excerpts followed by my interpretation;

"To be, or not to be, that is the question: Whether 'tis nobler in the mind to suffer The slings and arrows of outrageous fortune, Or to take arms against a sea of troubles And by opposing end them. To die—to sleep…To sleep, perchance to dream—ay, there's the rub: For in that sleep of death what dreams may come…But that the dread of something after death, makes us rather bear those ills we have Than fly to others that we know not of?" [24]

My interpretation:

'Should I live, or should I put myself out of my misery? Is it better to put up with the indiscriminate troubles and problems of life, or should I take matters into my own hands and end it all? Death; followed by nothingness. But here's the problem; maybe the 'sleep' of death is not oblivion or happy dreams; maybe it's a nightmare. Maybe it's worse than what I'm enduring now. And so the fear of what happens after death causes us to bear the troubles we have now rather than rush to others that we don't yet know about.

[22] CARL JUNG (PSYCHIATRIST AND COLLEAGUE OF SIGMUND FREUD).
[23] GILBERT M. BEEKEN
[24] WILLIAM SHAKESPEARE'S PLAY HAMLET, ACT 3, SCENE I.

For the first time since 1918 life expectancy in the United States is in decline. It was understandable that from 1915 to 1919 life expectancy declined because of World War 1, and the Spanish Flu Pandemic that killed 675,000 people in the United States. But in recent years life expectancy has been declining for very different reasons, drug overdoses and suicides.[25] That isn't a surprise when we are constantly being told that we are the product of random chance and we have no meaning or purpose. It's bleak and hopeless; people absolutely cannot live without meaning or purpose.

DESIGN

The Bible says, "The heavens proclaim the glory of God. The skies display his craftsmanship. Day after day they continue to speak; night after night they make Him known. They speak without a sound or word; their voice is never heard. Yet their message has gone throughout the earth and their words to all the world."[26] The famous American botanist, inventor and former slave, George Washington Carver said, "I like to think of nature as an unlimited radio

---

25

HTTPS://WWW.WASHINGTONPOST.COM/NATIONAL/HEALT H-SCIENCE/US-LIFE-EXPECTANCY-DECLINES-AGAIN-A-DISMAL-TREND-NOT-SEEN-SINCE-WORLD-WAR-1/2018/11/28/AE58BC8C-F28C-11E8-BC79-68604ED88993_STORY.HTML?UTM_TERM=.FDF94199A7EC
26 PSALM 19:1-5 (NLT)

station through which God speaks to us every hour, if we will only tune in."[27]

The Bible also says that "everyone knows the truth about God because He has made it obvious to them. For ever since the world was created, people have seen the earth and sky. Through everything God made, they can clearly see His invisible qualities—His eternal power and divine nature. So *they have no excuse for not knowing God.* Yes, they knew God, but they wouldn't worship Him as God or even give Him thanks."[28]

So according to the Bible, God has already clearly demonstrated His existence and His power by His creation. Creation doesn't tell us everything we need to know about God, but we can clearly see His creative power on display.

Every nation and people group in every century has had some concept of God; in fact religious people have always been and continue to be in the majority. They may not all believe in the same type of god, but they know there is someone powerful that put the earth together, because it's obvious.

There is just way too much evidence of design to think it could ever happen by random chance no matter how much time is allowed. When we see something as simple as rocks stacked into a column, we assume it is there by

[27]

HTTPS://WWW.BRAINYQUOTE.COM/QUOTES/GEORGE_WAS
HINGTON_CARVER_106884
[28] ROMANS 1: 18-21 (NLT)

design, stacked up by a person walking by and not stacked into a column by random chance over time.

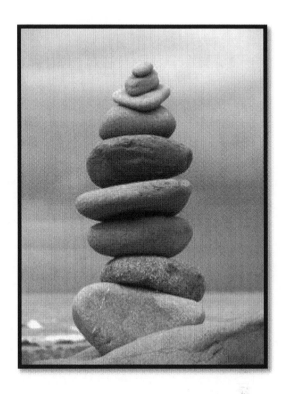

It would be difficult, but you might be able to stretch your imagination to believe that the rocks stacked up by chance if there was only one column of rocks. But if you saw numerous stacks of rocks, you would never draw that conclusion.

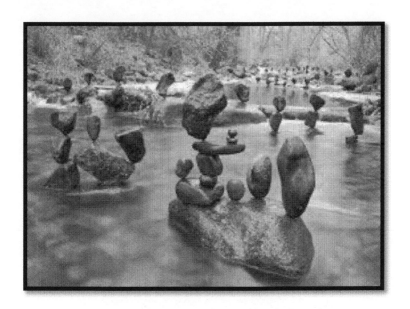

Rocks carefully balanced by design

There are countless examples of design; some are immense, like the solar system and galaxies. Some are so miniscule that they can only be seen with a microscope. They are all infinitely more complex than a handful of rocks stacked up.

Consider the cute little gecko with intricate feet that can walk on glass without sliding off. Researchers are investigating ways to create adhesives modeled on the feet of the gecko. [29]

[29] HTTPS://EN.WIKIPEDIA.ORG/WIKI/GECKO_FEET

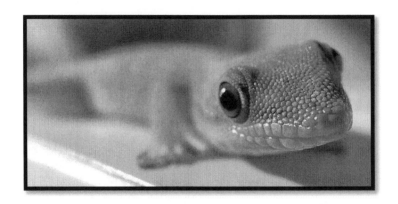

Gecko

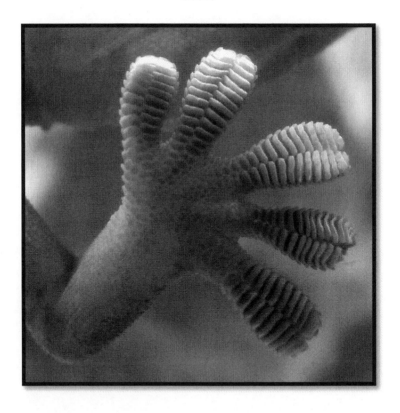

Gecko foot that can walk on glass. Their feet are even more astonishing when viewed at the microscopic level.

Then there is the tiny Bee Hummingbird that weighs less than 0.07 oz. or 2.0 g. and can hover in mid-air flapping its wings up to **80 times per second**! Some species of hummingbirds have been measured in wind tunnels, flying at speeds exceeding 34 mph, or 54 km/h. To conserve energy when sleeping or when food is scarce, they can go into torpor, a state similar to hibernation and slow their metabolic rate to $1/15^{th}$ of its normal rate. For hummingbirds to survive there are certain flowers that must also simultaneously be available to them for nutrients. One cannot evolve without the other, which only increases the complexity of design.[30]

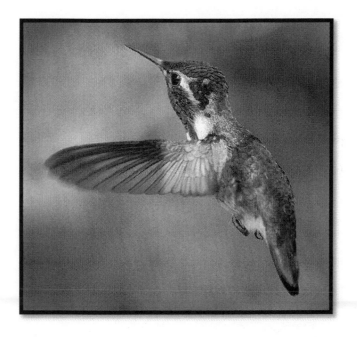

Bee Hummingbird

[30] HTTPS://EN.WIKIPEDIA.ORG/WIKI/HUMMINGBIRD

How about the Siberian willow warbler, such a small bird, but they are able to migrate at least 8,000 miles one way? Even more impressive perhaps is that they make the journey *alone* in their first year of life. *So since no other birds are going with them to show them the way, how do they know how to travel to a place 8,000 miles away?*

Researchers compared alternative compass routes with the routes the birds actually take. Based on this, they identified two alternative mechanisms that the willow warblers can use during their long migration — a solar compass that compensates for time shifts during the migration and a magnetic compass based on the assumption that the birds can measure the inclination angle of the Earth's magnetic field.[31] How does that miniscule bird brain know all of this? To me, that screams, "Design!"

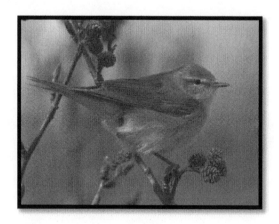

Siberian willow warbler

[31] WWW.SCI-NEWS.COM/BIOLOGY/SIBERIAN-WILLOW-WARBLERS-MIGRATION-06627.HTML

How is it that a giraffe can raise its head from ground level to the sky, some 15 feet up, and never get a head rush? "If we did that we'd certainly faint," says physiologist, Graham Mitchell of the University of Wyoming.[32] How could that evolve? The giraffe is either going to pass out, or it is not, there is no transitional form for that.

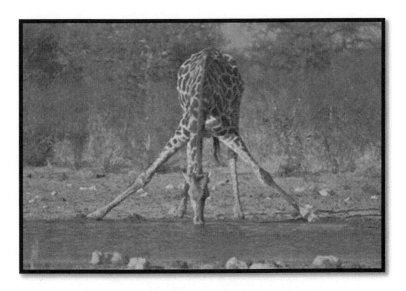

Then there is the cell; the smallest unit of life and the basic building block of all living things. There are trillions of cells in the human body providing structure for the body, taking in nutrients from food, converting those nutrients into energy, and carrying out specialized functions. Cells contain the body's hereditary material and can replicate themselves. [33]

---

[32] HTTPS://WWW.LIVESCIENCE.COM/853-GIRAFFES-DIZZY.HTML

[33] CELLHTTPS://GHR.NLM.NIH.GOV/PRIMER/BASICS/CELL

When Darwin came up with his evolutionary theory, little was known about the cell because the technology did not exist to study something so infinitesimal in sufficient detail. The cell was sort of a mystery and not thought to be nearly as complicated as we now know it to be. In fact, *each cell is actually an entire microscopic factory with very complex functions*.

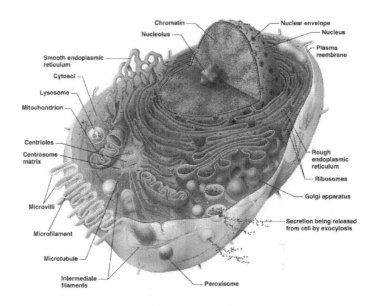

The parts of a single cell

One 'simple' cell is microscopic, and yet so complex that it seems like unbelievable science fiction! Located inside the nucleus of the cell is the DNA (Deoxyribonucleic acid) a molecule composed of two chains that coil around each other to form a double helix carrying the genetic instructions used in the growth, development, functioning and reproduction of all known organisms.[34]

"Some people think of the nucleus as the "brains" of the cell, but it is more like a hard disk. The nucleus stores all of the cell's important information. It stores our "code." Each of the cells in your body contains at least 20GB worth of information and there are almost 10 TRILLION cells in your body. The body stores its genetic information in an incredibly efficient manner. Our information technology has a long way to go before it matches the efficiency and capacity of the human body." [35]

In fact DNA's ability to store data is so incredible that; "…a group of researchers at the Swiss Federal Institute of Technology have found a way to encode data onto DNA— the very same stuff that all living beings' genetic information is stored on. One gram of DNA can potentially hold up to 455 exabytes of data, according to the New Scientist. For reference: There are one billion gigabytes in an exabyte, and 1,000 exabytes in a zettabyte. The cloud computing company EMC estimated that there were 1.8 zettabytes of data in the world in 2011, which means we would need only about 4 grams (about a teaspoon) of DNA to hold everything from Plato through the complete works of Shakespeare to Beyonce's latest album (not to mention every brunch photo ever posted on Instagram)."[36]

---

[34] HTTPS://EN.WIKIPEDIA.ORG/WIKI/DNA
[35] HTTP://WWW.MEDICINETHINK.COM/HOW-MUCH-DATA-IS-IN-A-CEL-POST-THANKSGIVING-FUN/
[36] HTTPS://QZ.COM/345640/SCIENTISTS-SAY-ALL-THE-WORLDS-DATA-CAN-FIT-ON-A-DNA-HARD-DRIVE-THE-SIZE-OF-A-TEASPOON/

Of all the evidences of design I can think of, the intricate functions accomplished by one single cell is the example that stuns me the most. One cell holds 20 GB of memory, and *one teaspoon of DNA can store all the information on the Internet 140 times over*! That is incredible! I'm sorry, but I am entirely incapable of believing that was not designed by a master engineer; random chance over unlimited time is completely out of the question. Keep in mind that the cell is not only incredibly complex, but it is also nanotechnology! There are just far too many 'stacked up rocks' for me to believe this is random. There is just much too much order. And just think; someone that powerful and intelligent values you so much!

The evidences of design are endless and I have only touched on a few that I found interesting. What about the human brain, the eye, the ear, nervous system, heart and circulatory system (which all have to be flawlessly functioning together at the very same time in order for the creature to survive at all)? Then there are the galaxies, the solar system, the water cycle, the oceans, diverse plants, and animals. All these things must function at the same time in order for any of us to survive. That's impossible!

Morris and I took a Botany class once where we learned that there is nothing simple about a leaf. Our professor periodically would literally jump up and down enthusiastically after explaining some complex aspect of plant life saying "Isn't that amazing?" Yes it is! *The more you know about any aspect of Creation, the more you realize its complexity and how unbelievable it is to think that any of it could ever happen by chance.* This is precisely why the Bible says, "Through everything God made, they can clearly see His invisible qualities—His eternal power and divine nature. So they have no excuse for not knowing God.[37]

We all take many things by faith; historical events or some scientific discoveries can only be taken by faith. For example, at the close of WWII in April 1945, American troops exposed the unspeakable atrocities of German concentration camps and the systematic slaughter of Jews and other innocent 'undesirables'. General Eisenhower said the following after exploring Buchenwald, "I visited every nook and cranny of the camp because I felt it my duty to be in a position from then on to testify at firsthand about these things in case there ever grew up at home the belief or assumption that 'the stories of Nazi brutality were just propaganda.'" [38]

He also ordered every soldier not at the immediate front to tour the camps in order for them to observe first-hand the evils and the cruelty inflicted on the Jews and other innocent prisoners. Eisenhower also arranged for various influential Americans and elected officials to see the evidence of the camps for themselves. The townspeople of Buchenwald were also compelled to view what they had allowed to happen next door. You have also probably seen many of the dreadful photos that were taken by American soldiers to document the evils they witnessed first-hand. Despite all the eye witnesses and overwhelming evidence

---

[37] ROMANS 1:20 (NLT)
[38] HTTPS://WWW.USHMM.ORG/EDUCATORS/TEACHING-MATERIALS/NATIONAL-HISTORY-DAY/RESEARCH-TOPICS/DWIGHT-D-EISENHOWER

they accumulated, there are people today who actually deny that it ever happened.[39]

Here's another example; in this day and age, one would assume that everyone knows and believes that the earth is round. Not so! Believe it or not there are some people who are still trying to convince us that the earth is flat. No doubt some of them are joking but there are plenty that are serious. They attribute the idea that the earth is round to some big cover-up and conspiracy, and have gone to great effort to attempt to convince the rest of us that the earth is flat, in spite of the data. [40]

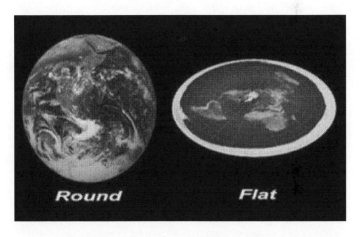

I was not even alive when the Allies discovered the barbaric occurrences at Buchenwald, but I believe it just the same (by faith) because of the testimony of so many eye witnesses and the evidence they collected.

---

[39] HTTPS://EN.WIKIPEDIA.ORG/WIKI/HOLOCAUST_DENIAL

[40] HTTPS://THEFLATEARTHSOCIETY.ORG/HOME/INDEX.PHP

I've never seen the earth from space and I have no way of determining for myself that the earth is round but I believe it (by faith) based on the evidence presented by other people who have done the research.   In both of these instances I believe something that I have not seen and could not see based on evidence presented by credible people. There is more than enough information to believe in the Holocaust and that the earth is round, but if someone will only believe what they can see and prove for themselves then there can never be enough proof for anything.

Since God has clearly revealed His existence, then no matter how much 'scientific' data is provided pro or con, at some point every person must decide by faith to believe in God or not. If someone doesn't want to believe in the face of all the evidence, then no amount of data will suffice because God has already provided the data.

PRAYER

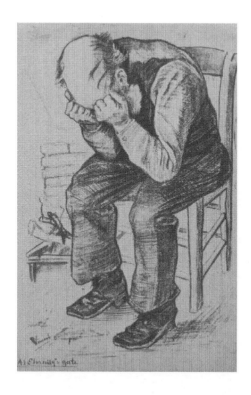

At Eternity's Gate by Vincent Van Gogh

I was surprised to learn that when he was a younger man, Vincent Van Gogh had been a Christian missionary to coal miners. He grew to admire the working poor and no doubt this drawing was inspired by one of those workers. Skye Jethani said "Looking at Van Gogh's drawing, I'm reminded that prayer is for the ordinary, simple and even the ignorant. It is for children and peasants, not just the pastors or the powerful." [41]

Prayer played a pivotal role in my fight with cancer; it made all the difference. I'm often surprised that I'm still alive when I think back on the whole catastrophic experience; I shouldn't be here, and I am firmly convinced that my recovery is due to prayer and God's miraculous intervention.

From the beginning of my battle with cancer I knew that many people were praying for me. Purcellville Baptist Church had my name in the bulletin as a prayer request throughout my entire struggle. Cornerstone Chapel had me on their prayer list, and sometimes quite unexpectedly people who hardly knew me told me they were praying for me daily!

A placebo is a harmless pill, medicine, or procedure prescribed more for the psychological benefit to the patient than for any physiological effect. Basically it doesn't do anything at all, good or bad. A placebo can be something as insignificant as a sugar pill. Even so, there have been cases where people were prescribed a placebo and their health actually improved. The explanation usually given for that is that the human body has the inherent ability in the immune system to heal itself, and somehow psychologically that ability is triggered or enhanced by the belief that the placebo is actually doing some good.

I know that some people regard prayer and/or faith as nothing more than a placebo. They would acknowledge that sometimes prayer appears to do some good, but they don't think it has any real benefit. In their minds prayer just gives people some sort of psychosomatic boost.

About 25 years ago I read of a scientific study of prayer and healing that recorded higher rates of recovery among people who were prayed for. An especially interesting finding of that particular study was that higher rates of recovery also occurred among people who did not even know they were being prayed for, which would eliminate the placebo effect. Unfortunately I have not been able to find that old study but I am just mentioning that it exists in case you have an interest in looking into it.

But with or without that study, ultimately belief in God and that He answers prayer comes down to faith. A good illustration of this is a Reader's Digest article I read many years ago, I think it was 1976. I don't remember the title but it was a true story about a man who was swept overboard off a ship one night off the coast of Miami, Florida. Floating in the dark water, he could see the distant skyline of Miami, much too far away to swim to. No ships were around, and who would see or hear him in the dark water even if a ship did happen by? His situation was hopeless, in his own estimation.

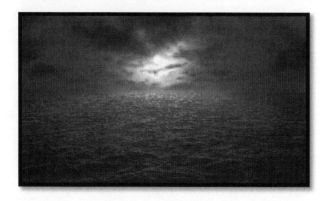

The man was an agnostic, but in his desperation he prayed. He told God he did not know if He even existed, but if He did he asked Him to rescue him. Not long after, a ship passed by, miraculously they were able to hear him, and fished him out of the dark water! Unfortunately, (but somewhat predictably) the man's conclusion was this, "I'll never know if that was Divine Intervention, or just luck."

I remember rolling my eyes and thinking "you've got to be kidding." If people do not want to acknowledge God or His aid, no amount of empirical evidence will ever suffice.

PAIN AND SUFFERING

"Pain insists upon being attended to. God whispers to us in our pleasures, speaks in our consciences, but shouts in our pains. It is his megaphone to rouse a deaf world."
— C.S. Lewis [42]

The Bible is full of what Christians call 'Precious Promises.' We'd prefer promises of continuous peace, prosperity and happiness. But Jesus promised, "Here on earth you will have many trials and sorrows. But take heart, because I have overcome the world."[43] So even when life seems to be completely out of control and everything is falling apart, Jesus told us that he is with us and has overcome the world. He is stronger than us and is

---

[42]
HTTP://THINKEXIST.COM/QUOTATION/GOD_WHISPERS_TO _US_IN_OUR_PLEASURES-SPEAKS_TO_US/180233.HTML
[43] JOHN 16:33 (NLT)

in control of our lives even when things appear to have gone all wrong. That is another reason why I was able to have peace in the middle of my life and death health crisis.

The Bible also says that "our present troubles are small and won't last very long. Yet they produce for us a glory that vastly outweighs them and will last forever!"[44] Our present troubles often appear enormous and insurmountable, and can seem unbearable and interminable, but the Bible states just the opposite. They are 'light' and 'won't last very long' when compared with the weighty blessings we will experience without end.

One especially difficult aspect of suffering is that it often feels random and pointless, but for believers our sufferings are never pointless. They are 'producing for us a glory that vastly outweighs them and will last forever.' When things are going well we don't tend to reflect or think too deeply about the big questions; we just coast along in comfort and bliss. But suffering and trouble compel us to ponder and ask the hard questions that sometimes don't appear to have good answers. Suffering changes us. Helen Keller, the first deaf and blind person to earn a Bachelor of Arts degree said, "We would never learn to be brave or patient if there were only joy in the world."[45]

Suffering makes some people stronger and better while others become hardened and bitter over painful circumstances. They become filled with anger and self-pity. Suffering can make us better, or bitter depending on how we respond to it. The following two Biblical

---

[44] 2 CORINTHIANS 4:17 (NLT)
[45]
HTTPS://WWW.BRAINYQUOTE.COM/QUOTES/HELEN_KELLE
R_385215

characters suffered enormously, but they did not become bitter or hard.

JOSEPH

Joseph endured 14 long years of suffering; his story begins in Genesis 37. Joseph's father, Jacob, had 12 sons. Joseph's family was extremely dysfunctional; his father, Jacob, favored Joseph above all his brothers and they all knew it. Joseph had a couple of dreams and told his brothers about them. Both dreams predicted that Joseph would eventually rule over his brothers. Hearing about Joseph's dreams made his brothers even angrier, if that's possible. Then his father tangibly demonstrated his favoritism toward Joseph by giving him an extremely expensive multi-colored robe, but none to his brothers, which only increased his brothers' jealousy and rage.

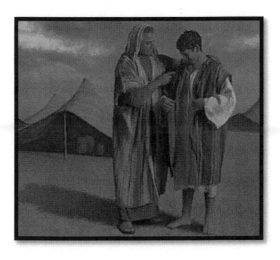

One day Joseph's father directed him to go check up on his brothers as they tended sheep in the countryside. When his brothers saw Joseph approaching in the distance they saw it as a golden opportunity to get rid of him once and for all. They hated him so much that they originally planned to kill him. But when a caravan of merchants heading for Egypt passed by they seized the opportunity to get rid of Joseph and make a little money at the same time. Ignoring Joseph's cries for mercy; they sold their brother, Joseph, into slavery. They weren't just having a weak moment. They knew exactly what they were doing and they did it intentionally. Then they lied to their father, Jacob, and told him that Joseph had been killed by a wild animal. Jacob was devastated.

In Egypt Joseph became the property of an Egyptian officer named Potiphar. Because he had such excellent administrative skills, before long Joseph was entrusted with managing Potiphar's entire estate. Joseph was a very handsome young man and Potiphar's wife repeatedly attempted to seduce him. He resisted her advances but one day she found him alone in the house and Joseph's only way of escape was to run out of the house, leaving his robe in her hands. She falsely accused him of attempted rape, presenting his robe as evidence and Joseph was thrown into prison.

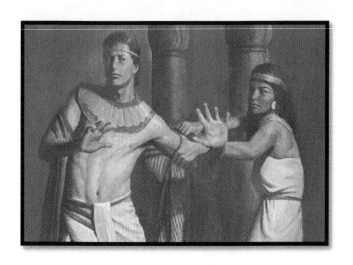

Joseph fleeing from Potiphar's wife

Even in prison Joseph's administrative skills served him well. The warden soon put the entire prison under his management. Two political prisoners, (the Pharaoh's cup-bearer and baker) both had distressing dreams and with God's help Joseph was able to accurately foresee what the dreams meant and what would happen to each of the prisoners. Just as Joseph predicted, the baker was executed and the cup-bearer was reinstated to his position, but he promptly forgot all about Joseph.

Two more years passed and then the Pharaoh had two disturbing dreams that no one could interpret. Finally the cup-bearer remembered that Joseph had correctly interpreted his dream and he told Pharaoh that Joseph could tell him what his dreams meant. Joseph was summoned and again with God's help he accurately interpreted the meaning of Pharaoh's dreams. He told Pharaoh that the dreams meant that there would be 7 years of plenty followed by 7 years of severe famine. He recommended a wise course of action in response to this bad news. The Pharaoh was so impressed by his advice that he appointed Joseph to be second-in-command in Egypt! Only the Pharaoh himself would be more powerful than Joseph!

The 7 years of plenty were followed by 7 years of famine just as Joseph predicted. Because of his prudent preparations, storing up grain during the years of plenty, the Egyptians had more than enough to eat, and plenty left over to sell to the surrounding tribes and nations. The extreme famine finally forced Jacob to send his sons to Egypt to buy grain. Joseph was in charge of the grain and recognized his brother's immediately when they came to him to purchase grain, but they did not recognize Joseph. He was older now and he dressed and spoke like an Egyptian. They expected that Joseph probably would dead by that time and they could never have guessed that instead he was the second most powerful man in Egypt! Joseph was now ruling over his brothers just as his earlier dreams had foretold.

While his brothers still did not know who he was, Joseph put them through a few tests to determine if their hard hearts had softened over the years, before revealing his identity to them. They didn't know it but Joseph understood them and he heard them speaking among themselves. They said, "Clearly we are being punished because of what we did to Joseph long ago. We saw his anguish when he pleaded for his life, but we wouldn't listen. That's why we're in this trouble."[46] Eventually Joseph returned to his father, Jacob, with wagons, to bring him and his entire extended family of 77 persons back to Egypt. There they were treated as honored guests of the

---

[46] GENESIS 42:21 (NLT)

Pharaoh. When Jacob died he was mourned by the Egyptians.

After their father died, Joseph's brothers were terrified that Joseph would finally take his revenge on them for all the wrong they had done to him. So they sent this message to Joseph: "Before your father died, he instructed us to say to you: 'Please forgive your brothers for the great wrong they did to you—for their sin in treating you so cruelly.' So we, the servants of the God of your father, beg you to forgive our sin." When Joseph received the message, he broke down and wept. Then his brothers came and threw themselves down before Joseph. "Look, we are your slaves!" they said. [47]

But Joseph replied, "Don't be afraid of me. Am I God, that I can punish you? *You intended to harm me, but God intended it all for good.* He brought me to this position so I could save the lives of many people. No, don't be afraid. I will continue to take care of you and your children." So he reassured them by speaking kindly to them. [48]

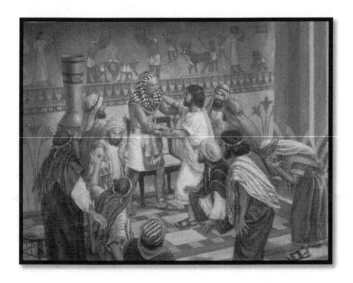

[47] GENESIS 50:16-18 (NLT)
[48] GENESIS 50:19-21 (NLT)

Joseph experienced the prolonged pain and suffering of being rejected by his family, betrayed by his brothers, sold as a slave, then falsely accused and imprisoned. He spent 14 long years suffering unjustly before ultimately becoming the second most powerful person in Egypt. In Joseph's own words he acknowledged that his brothers intended to harm him; it was intentional evil. But God intended it for good to save the lives of many people. *Only God can bring genuine good from absolute evil.*

'God causes everything to work together for the good of those who love God and are called according to his purpose for them.'[49] That does not mean that everything that happens to a believer is actually good. It means that God will take situations and occurrences that truly are bad and bring genuine good from them whether they are unfortunate random accidents or intentional malicious assaults. For the Christian, our suffering is never pointless or wasted. I still don't really know why the whole 'cancer thing' happened to me, but it's not pointless. For one thing it has changed my perspective on many things. This book may even be a reason because I would never have written it otherwise.

A question that is almost always asked when bad things happen is "Why?" One bad thing after another happened to Joseph, but in time he was able to see how all those terrible experiences positioned him to be in the right place at the right time. Having a relationship with God and knowing that He is involved and in complete control is what enables us to have peace, even when events seem like uncontrollable accidents or random coincidences.

---

[49] ROMANS 8:28 (NLT)

Joseph lived to see and understand how God used his suffering for great good, saving the lives of his immediate family as well as many others. But that's not always how it happens. Sometimes we never know why, as was the case for Job.

JOB

God Himself said that Job was a good man. He was also the wealthiest man in his region. He had 10 children, vast herds and many servants. He had a reputation as a wise and good man who generously helped the poor. The book of Job tells us that one day the members of the heavenly court came to present themselves before the Lord, and the Accuser, Satan came with them. "Where have you come from?" the Lord asked Satan. Satan answered the Lord, "I have been patrolling the earth, watching everything that's going on."

Then the Lord asked Satan, "Have you noticed my servant Job? He is the finest man in all the earth. He is blameless—a man of complete integrity. He fears God and stays away from evil."

Satan replied to the Lord, "Yes, but Job has good reason to fear (reverence) God. You have always put a wall of protection around him and his home and his property. You have made him prosper in everything he does. Look how rich he is! But reach out and take away everything he has and he will surely curse you to your face!"

"All right, you may test him," the Lord said to Satan. "Do whatever you want with everything he possesses, but don't harm him physically." So Satan left the Lord's presence. [50] In very short order all of Job's livestock were stolen and a strong wind blew down the house where Job's children had been feasting, killing them all instantly. Even so, Job said, "I came naked from my mother's womb, and I will be naked when I leave. The Lord gave me what I had, and the Lord has taken it away. Praise the name of the Lord!" In all of this, Job did not sin by blaming God. [51]

Since that didn't work, Satan asked permission to attack Job's health to get him to curse God. It's interesting that he had to ask permission, but God granted it. That is a strong indicator that nothing happens to God's children that God does not allow for His purposes. Even if things look bad, we do not know the rest of the story. We've all had the experience of hearing one side of a story. We can become indignant and want to take action on behalf of the injured party. Then when we hear the other side of the story and get a few more facts our opinion might change entirely. We cannot see the big picture; we never have all the facts, but God does. That's where faith and trust comes in.

Job's story only got worse; he got sick and even his wife suggested that he should just 'curse God and die.' She had shared Job's losses and had gone from being the most prestigious woman in the area to being penniless and a target of ridicule and humiliation. Maybe she figured her

---

[50] JOB 1:6-12 (NLT)

[51] JOB 1:21-22 (NLT)

own situation would improve if Job was gone. In any case, Job's wife was no help.

Job's friends came to comfort him and were speechless when they first saw his horrifying condition. Eventually they came to the conclusion that all this suffering would never happen to a good person. Job must have secretly done something terrible to bring all this pain and misery on himself and they tried to get him to admit it. So rather than encouraging their friend, Job, they accused him of concealing unconfessed wickedness. Not only had he lost everything, but he also lost the support of everyone. They all thought that Job was only getting what he deserved.

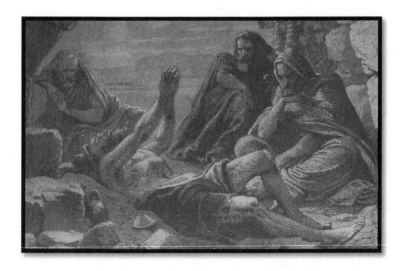

Job and his friends who were 'miserable comforters'

We know that God Himself said that Job was the finest man in all the earth. He was blameless—a man of complete integrity. He feared God and stayed away from evil. That is God's assessment of Job, so we know that he was not getting what he deserved. *It was a case of bad things happening to good people.*

Job questioned why all these terrible things happened to him. "Why?" He was a regular human like we are and it's only natural to wonder. We hate to think that our suffering is meaningless, accidental or out of control. We know for certain that Job did nothing to deserve what happened to him, but he never learned why any of it happened, not in this life anyway.

In the end God did not tell Job what caused his sufferings, but God restored Job's wealth, in fact he doubled it. Job also had 10 more children (presumably the other 10 children were in heaven and he hadn't really lost them either). Throughout all of his sorrows, Job did not curse or blame God. In fact in the middle of all his suffering he stated, "Though he slay me, yet will I trust him."[52] Suffering did not make Job bitter.

---

[52] JOB 13:15 (NLT)

CHAPTER 8

FAITH ALONE

Faith in God can certainly help with recovery from health problems and make life better in this present world. But even if my faith in God helped me live to 120 years old in perfect health, that would still be insignificant when compared to eternity. What gave me such peace in the middle of my near death experience is my faith that my life now and forever is in God's hands. Even if I die (and I will still die someday) I will have everlasting life in heaven with God. So I cannot lose either way. As Paul the apostle said, "For to me, to live is Christ and to die is gain." [53]

Today many believe that all it takes to get into heaven is to die. In other words, everyone goes to heaven. It's part of the myth that people are basically good, which is a humanist position. Humanism, a common worldview in our culture today, is a system of thought that relies on human strength and intellect rather than divine or supernatural power for problem solving. Humanists stress the basic goodness of human beings. This worldview is so pervasive today that even many Christians believe that humankind is basically good.

But the Bible says that, "God saw that the wickedness of man was great in the earth, and that *every imagination of*

---

[53] PHILIPPIANS 1:21 (NLT)

the thoughts of his heart was <u>only</u> <u>evil</u> <u>continually</u>."[54]
God said, "Everything they think or imagine is bent toward evil from childhood"[55] "The human heart is the most deceitful of all things, and desperately wicked. Who really knows how bad it is?" [56] "There is none righteous, no, not one,"[57] which excludes everyone! The Bible very clearly teaches that the heart of the human problem is the human heart. [58]

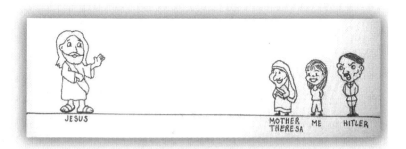

The theologian, R.C. Sproul illustrated this for his seminary students by asking one of them to stand at the far left side of the classroom representing Jesus. A notorious villain, such as Hitler was represented by another student standing on the far right. The rest of the class was asked to take a position between the perfection of Jesus and the wickedness of Hitler based on their evaluation of their own morality. Mostly they selected positions in the center, but Dr. Sproul explained that to be Biblically accurate they should all be standing next to Hitler. We're not even close to the righteousness of Jesus.

---

[54] GENESIS 6:5 (NLT)
[55] GENESIS 8:21 (NLT)
[56] JEREMIAH 17:9 (NLT)
[57] ROMANS 3:10 (NLT)
[58]
HTTPS://CORNERSTONECHAPEL.NET/?PAGE_ID=418&I=1348

The Bible tells us that God created everything, including the first human beings; Adam and Eve. He provided them with a beautiful garden (Eden) to live in that had everything they needed; a perfect environment filled with a wide variety of fruits. Adam and Eve were intended to rule the earth with God and in fellowship (friendship) with Him.

There was only one tree in the middle of the garden that they were told not to eat of; the Tree of the Knowledge of Good and Evil, and if they were ever to eat of it they would die. There was only the one very easy law to keep; not to eat from one tree out of thousands. God always wanted a voluntary, loving relationship with human kind. He did not want robots that were compelled to love and obey Him. So God gave them freedom of choice. There was only one law, and they could freely choose whether to obey it and enjoy immortality, joy, life and peace; or choose to do their own thing.

People often debate what causes bad character; is it nature, or nurture? Are people just naturally born with a predisposition toward good or bad behavior because of their individual genetics (their nature)? Or is it because of the environment they were raised in, such as the good or bad examples set by their parents, teachers and friends; or by difficult life experiences such as poverty, war or crime (nurture)? It might be a little bit of both, but whatever the cause, Adam and Eve did not have any of those handicaps or excuses. They did not have any inherited defects, and they had always lived in a perfect environment. They were in the best possible position to have the character to do the right thing in every circumstance.

But despite having every possible advantage they quickly yielded to temptation and broke the only law there was; don't eat from the Tree of the Knowledge of Good and Evil. They chose to defy God, not wanting to rule in companionship with God. They chose to be apart from Him and assume a position of control. That single act of disobedience shattered Adam and Eve's relationship with God and each other, and death and suffering entered the world. [59]

We are all born with a sinful nature and not inclined to obey or seek after God. We are defiant rebels against God, and proud of it. God has not offended us, He is the offended party. And yet, God is the one who took the initiative to restore our relationship with Him. "For the sin of this one man, Adam, brought death to many. But even greater is God's wonderful grace and His gift of forgiveness to many through this other man, Jesus Christ."[60] We human beings were not particularly interested in restoring the relationship, and we couldn't do it even if we tried.

The world is not what God originally intended it to be. Because of humankind's rebellion it has become a scary place filled with pain, disease, dangerous natural disasters, conflict and scarce resources among other things. Religions originate from mankind's fear and desire to gain control over things that are far beyond our control. We try to do favors for God to manipulate and obligate Him to act on our behalf thinking, 'if I do this, then God will do that.' It is an attempt to put God in our debt and force Him to do our bidding. But the God of the Bible is not the kind of

---

[59] GENESIS CHAPTERS 2-3 (NLT)
[60] ROMANS 5:15 (NLT)

God anyone would invent. He is completely unmanageable. It's true that we often think of God as a butler or therapist, but He is neither. ***What God seeks, and has always sought is a loving relationship with us.***

Most of us are able to conceal and not act upon every bad thought or impulse we have. But we know that we would be humiliated if people could read our minds and all our thoughts or if all our thoughts were broadcast on CNN. The Bible describes God as all knowing (omniscient), all powerful (omnipotent), and present in all places at all times (omnipresent). He knows all our thoughts, but loves us anyway. The One who knows us best, loves us most (even with what He knows!) Incredible!

The 1997 movie, Liar, Liar, starring Jim Carrey illustrated this truth in an amusing way. Jim Carrey's character was a notorious liar. He became unable to lie for a full 24 hours after his son's birthday wish came true; that his dad would tell the truth. Carrey had to tell the truth in every situation, at all times. So if he hated a woman's dress or hairstyle or thought she was fat and ugly, he told her exactly what he thought. When he tried to make up excuses for missing his son's game or being late for work or an appointment, instead he was compelled to admit the truth.

Obviously, always telling the exact truth about what is going on inside our heads would be disastrous. That's because we are not basically good. We have just learned to rein in most of our bad behavior. Some people succeed at that better than others, but nobody does it perfectly, and the standard is perfection.

That's what Jesus said; "But you are to be perfect, even as your Father in heaven is perfect."[61] If that's true we are all in serious trouble, because nobody is perfect, in fact we are not even close! No one has to teach their sweet, innocent children how to lie or disobey. It comes naturally; we have to train them to tell the truth, not to cheat or steal, and to share their toys. People are not basically, inherently good.

Another myth is that God grades on the curve. It's the idea that if I behave better than most other people that's good enough. The cut off for excessively bad behavior is always somewhere just below me. The tendency is to compare ourselves with other people. We choose someone really terrible like Hitler and compared to him we think we look really great. We all know we're not nearly as selfless and self-sacrificing as someone like Mother Teresa, but we're a whole lot better than Hitler so we figure that's good enough. We may appear morally superior compared to other people, but the problem is that we are comparing ourselves to the wrong people. They are not the standard. The standard is the sinless perfection of Jesus. When compared to Jesus, we all fall miserably short.

Christianity is unique when compared to other religions. Other religions seek to gain God's acceptance by their good deeds, hard work, self-denial, rituals, and sacrifices. Christianity is different. It is God reaching down to help us and doing for us what we never could do for ourselves. Man could not reach up to God. To think that is possible one must reduce God, make Him less, and at the same time increase oneself. So God sent His Son to lift us up and reconcile us to Himself; to make peace between us

---

[61] MATTHEW 5:48 (NLT)

and Him, *doing for us what we could never do for ourselves.*

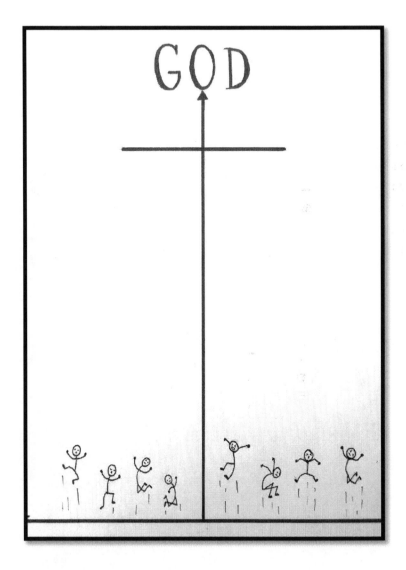

Some people may give the appearance of growing closer to God's standard of perfection by their good deeds and devotion. But even our very best efforts fall pitifully short; according to the Bible, no one is 'good enough', not even one.

We all know we've done wrong, either intentionally or unintentionally. But our situation is a whole lot worse than we think and this is why. One of the 10 Commandments is "You must not be envious of your neighbor's house, or want to sleep with his wife, or want to own his slaves, oxen, donkeys, or anything else he has.'"[62] The thing to notice here is that *to be envious (jealous, covetous) is not an action; it is an attitude or a thought.* Someone may envy or be jealous of their neighbor's car, but that's much different than actually stealing it. But God knows all our attitudes and thoughts, and they count against us even if we don't act on them. Here is another example; Jesus said, "Anyone who hates (an attitude) another brother or sister is really a murderer at heart. And you know that murderers don't have eternal life within them."[63]

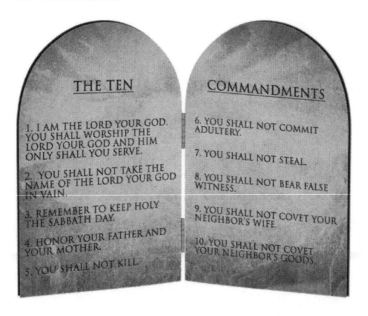

The Ten Commandments

---

[62] EXODUS 5:17 (NLT)
[63] 1 JOHN 3:15 (NLT)

Jesus said, "You have heard the commandment that says, 'You must not commit adultery.' But I say, anyone who even looks at a woman with lust has already committed adultery with her in his heart."[64] *God is just as interested in our motives, as He is in our actions*, and often our motives are self-centered even though our actions appear honorable. "The LORD does not look at the things people look at. People look at the outward appearance, but the LORD looks at the heart."[65]

God is a lot smarter than we are. He knows everything we have done, but He also knows our thoughts and our thoughts matter as much to Him as our actions. When our thoughts and motivations are factored in, our situation becomes catastrophic. We are much guiltier than we think. We can't change ourselves, but He said He will. "For God is working in you, giving you the desire and the power to do what pleases Him." [66]

Another common myth is that we can improve our dismal condition and earn a few extra points with God all by ourselves, by our good deeds. Everyone knows that 'nobody is perfect'. That's often the first comment out of our mouth if someone criticizes our actions. We all know that we are imperfect, but we feel we're not all that bad compared to everybody else (in our own opinion). We can trick ourselves into believing that we just need to do a few extra good deeds or stop doing a few bad habits to make up the difference and balance things out in our favor.

But there are problems with that. Even if from this moment on you lived a perfect life, what about the things

---

[64] MATTHEW 5:27-28 (NLT)
[65] I SAMUEL 16:7 (NLT)
[66] PHILIPPIANS 2:13 (NLT)

you have already done? They don't magically disappear just because you've changed your ways any more than a very nice repentant murderer or thief who promises never to do it again would be freed from prison. It doesn't work like that. You do the crime, you do the time. Any judge that issued acquittals without punishment for crimes would be unjust, and God is not unjust.

There was an ancient Jewish sect at Jesus' time called the Pharisees who were distinguished by strict observance of the traditional and written law. They thought of themselves as more righteous than everyone else because they worked so hard at obeying even the tiniest detail of the Law. Such a person today would be called self-righteous, or a hypocrite.

Jesus welcomed everyone and was patient and kind even when interacting with society's outcasts such as prostitutes and hated tax collectors. In those days tax collectors were Jews who worked for the Romans collecting taxes. They were viewed as traitors because they made a lavish income out of overcharging the people. Basically they were thieves.

But Jesus generally had tough words for the Pharisees. They looked good on the outside, making a good show of being self-controlled making long prayers in public, avoiding sensual matters, yet they were seething with hidden worldly desires. They were full of greed and self-indulgence and their veneer of righteousness hid a secret inner world of ungodly thoughts and feelings. They were full of wickedness. Jesus said they 'were like whitewashed tombs, beautiful on the outside, but full of dead men's bones.'[67]

The Pharisees are the quintessential example of trying to please God based on one's own good efforts, and Jesus said to them, "You are of your father, the Devil."[68] Offering God our very best efforts does not turn out well; our very best efforts are not nearly good enough. Until we understand this bad news, we don't know how much we need the good news.

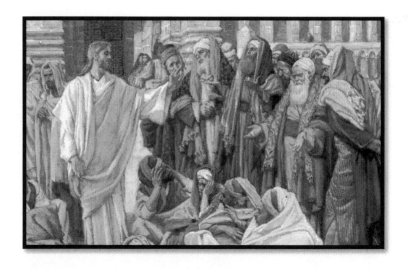

Jesus and the Pharisees

God really does want to pardon and make peace with us though, that's the good news, and He made it very easy for us. ***God did all the work and we do none of it.*** Our salvation is not the result of any of our efforts, abilities,

[67] MATTHEW 23:27 (NLT)
[68] JOHN 8:44 (NLT)

intelligent choices, personal characteristics, or acts of service we may perform. "God saved you by His grace when you believed. And you can't take credit for this; it is a gift from God. *Salvation is not a reward for the good things we have done, so none of us can boast about it.*" [69]

When I was a kid I often turned on the TV after school to watch old movies. Some of my favorites were jungle adventures, like "Tarzan." Once in a while some unsuspecting traveler trudging through the jungle stepped into quicksand and quickly began to sink. The more he struggled, the faster he sank, and before long he dropped out of sight.

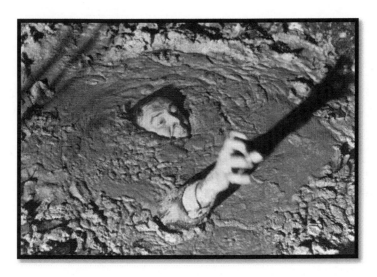

Sinking in quicksand

Actually, your body will float in quicksand if you just relax, but it is true that the more you struggle in it the faster you will sink. Therefore, you cannot get out of quicksand without help. In the same way, we cannot dig

---

[69] EPHESIANS 2:9 (NLT)

ourselves out of the pit of sin that we all have fallen into, no matter how much we struggle. But God wants very much to lift us out; "He lifted me out of the slimy pit, out of the mud and mire; He set my feet on a rock and gave me a firm place to stand."[70]

God would not be just and righteous to ignore our sins and let them go unpunished. But we are powerless to set things right either. We cannot undo our sins by doing good deeds. "When we were utterly helpless, Christ came at just the right time and died for us sinners. Now, most people would not be willing to die for an upright person, though someone might perhaps be willing to die for a person who is especially good. But God showed his great love for us by sending Christ to die for us while we were still sinners."[71]

If Christ had sinned, then he would also be guilty and could not help us. He "understands our weaknesses, for he faced all of the same testings we do, yet he did not sin." [72] Since he was innocent and perfect he could voluntarily take on our punishment, in the same way that a wealthy person could choose to pay off the crushing debt of a poor person. Someone who can pay is able to pay off a debt for someone who cannot.

"Every time we look at the cross, Christ seems to be saying to us, 'I am here because of you. It is your sin I am bearing, your curse I am suffering, your debt I am paying, your death I am dying.' Nothing in all of history or the universe cuts us down to size like the cross. All of us have

---

[70] PSALM 40:2 (NLT)
[71] ROMANS 5:7-8 (NLT)
[72] HEBREWS 4:15 (NLT)

201

inflated views of ourselves, especially in self-righteousness, until we visit a place called Calvary. It is there, at the foot of the cross that we shrink to our true size."[73] We owed a debt we could not pay. Jesus paid a debt he did not owe.

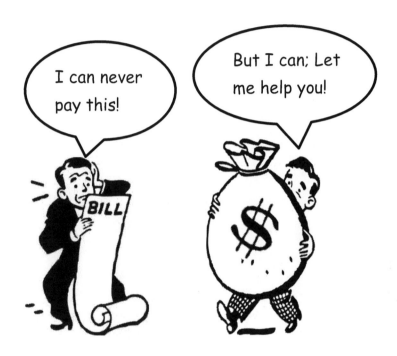

Jesus said "no one can take my life from me. I sacrifice it voluntarily."[74] He also said, "There is no greater love than to lay down one's life for one's friends."[75]

When the soldiers came to take Jesus away to be crucified, Peter, one of his disciples, pulled out a sword to defend

73
HTTPS://WORLDLYSAINTS.WORDPRESS.COM/2015/05/03/JO
HN-STOTT-ON-HOW-THE-CROSS-HUMBLES-US/
[74] JOHN 10:18
[75] JOHN 15:13

him and cut off a man's ear. Jesus healed the man's ear and told Peter to put away his sword. Jesus said, "Don't you realize that I could ask my Father for thousands of angels to protect us and He would send them instantly? But if I did, how would the Scriptures be fulfilled that describe what must happen now?"[76]

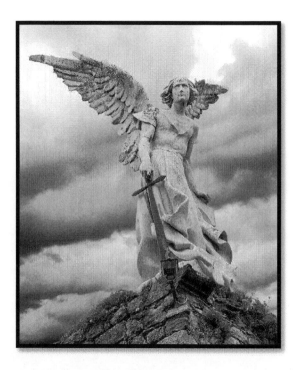

Angels are not like cute little babies with wings as some artists portray them. They are powerful and intimidating, and when humans have encountered them they always cower in fear.

It's interesting to note that 1) Jesus voluntarily chose to die for our sins, in our place, and that He had the power,

---

[76] MATTHEW 26:53-54

[76] MATTHEW 26:53-54

203

even at the last minute, to wipe out anyone who tried to kill him. In 2 Kings 19:35 one angel alone is reported to have killed 185,000 men, so having thousands of angels at his disposal made Jesus invincible. He chose to die in our place. Jesus said, "No one can take my life from me. I sacrifice it voluntarily. For I have the authority to lay it down when I want to and also to take it up again. For this is what my Father has commanded."[77] 2) His death was predicted long before. Jesus fulfilled over 300 very specific prophesies in the Bible. Jesus even predicted events before he was crucified, saying; "I have told you these things before they happen so that when they do happen, you will believe."[78]

What if I told you that you would find a lottery ticket today and that in three days you would win the lottery and you would book passage on a cruise around the world on the Princess Cruise Line, and that they would randomly assign you room number 213? And then I also predicted that exactly 10 days later when the ship was 250 miles from Hawaii a helicopter would come to make an emergency evacuation of a heart patient named Michelangelo Albergeti. If all of that actually happened in that exact time frame I'm guessing that would get your attention.

You could control whether or not you book a cruise, but nobody could control the rest of that! Going back to the story of Joseph, God helped him interpret the prophetic meanings of the prisoner's dreams and Pharaoh's dreams. Events transpired exactly as he said they would, which is one of the reasons he had so much credibility.

---

[77] JOHN 10:18 (NLT)
[78] JOHN 14:29 (NLT)

God is outside of time and can see the end and the beginning all at once. He says, "Only I can tell you the future before it even happens. Everything I plan will come to pass, for I do whatever I wish."[79]

According to Dr. Peter W. Stoner, mathematically, the odds that Jesus would fulfill just 8 of the more than 300 prophecies about him are: 1 in 100,000,000,000,000,000. Just one prophesy for example was that he would be born in Bethlehem . The number of people who have ever been born in Bethlehem is relatively small so this already eliminates most of the people who have ever been born or ever will be. But Mary and Joseph were from Nazareth, 90 miles away, and she was 9 months pregnant! As it happened, Caesar Augustus decided that would be a good time to require his subjects to return to their ancestral homes to register to be taxed. Mary and Joseph were forced to take that long trip at the worst possible time, arriving just in time for Jesus to be born in Bethlehem. A baby could not control where he would be born, but God made sure to get Jesus' mother to Bethlehem just in time for his birth!

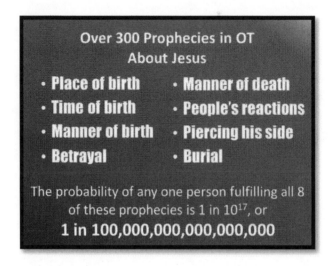

Over 300 Prophecies in OT
About Jesus

- **Place of birth**
- **Time of birth**
- **Manner of birth**
- **Betrayal**

- **Manner of death**
- **People's reactions**
- **Piercing his side**
- **Burial**

The probability of any one person fulfilling all 8 of these prophecies is 1 in 10^{17}, or
1 in 100,000,000,000,000,000

[79] ISAIAH 46:10 (NLT)

For one person to fulfill 48 of the prophecies would be: 1 chance in 10 to the 157th power. That's a number far too large to even contemplate, but there are not just 48 prophesies about Jesus, there are over 300!

Josh McDowell was preparing to be a lawyer. He was an agnostic at college when he decided to compose a paper that would examine the historical evidence of the Christian faith. He did this for the expressed purpose of disproving Christianity. However, he converted to Christianity after, as he says, he found evidence for it, not against it.[80] Instead of refuting Christianity he became a Christian and authored the book, Evidence that Demands a Verdict to lay out the evidence.

Lee Strobel has a journalism degree and a law degree from Yale, and was a journalist for the Chicago Tribune and other newspapers for 14 years. Lee states he was an atheist when he began investigating the Biblical claims about Christ after his wife became a Christian. He expected to expose it as false. Instead, prompted by the results of his investigation he became a Christian in 1981, and subsequently, a pastor. He also authored the book, The Case for Christ.

Dr. Simon Greenleaf helped establish Harvard Law School and wrote the legal masterpiece, *A Treatise on the Law of Evidence*, which is still in use today. He decided to put Jesus' resurrection on trial by examining the evidence. As a legal scholar, Greenleaf wondered if Jesus' resurrection would meet his stringent tests for evidence and whether or not the evidence for it would hold up in a court of law. Focusing his brilliant legal mind on the facts of history, Greenleaf began applying his rules of evidence to the case of Jesus' resurrection.

---

[80] JOSH MCDOWELL, EVIDENCE THAT DEMANDS A VERDICT

Contrary to what skeptics might have expected, the more Greenleaf investigated the record of history, the more evidence he discovered supporting the claim that Jesus had indeed risen from the tomb.[81] Greenleaf concluded that, "According to the laws of legal evidence used in courts of law, there is more evidence for the historical fact of the resurrection of Jesus Christ than for just about any other event in history." He also said, *A person who rejects Christ may choose to say that I do not accept it, he may not choose to say there is not enough evidence."* [82]

It often happens that people who seriously attempt to refute the claims of Christianity end up becoming convinced that it is true, and convert to Christianity. Like the Police Cold-Case Investigator, J. Warner Wallace who turned to Science to disprove Christ's resurrection, and got shocked by the evidence. Instead he became a Christian and wrote the book, Cold-Case Christianity .

Chuck Colson, Special Counsel (legal counsel) to President Nixon was also prompted to examine the truth claims and evidence for Christianity from a legal standpoint after a friend gave him a copy of Mere Christianity. He concluded it was true which led him to become a Christian. Colson subsequently wrote the book, Born Again about how he became a Christian, and founded a Christian ministry to prisoners, called Prison Fellowship. As it happens Prison Fellowship is where Morris worked for most of his career. Colson devoted the remainder of his life to sharing his faith with prisoners.

---

[81] HTTPS://Y-JESUS.COM/SIMON-GREENLEAF-RESURRECTION/
[82] HTTPS://WWW.QUORA.COM/WHAT-ARE-THE-BEST-QUOTES-FROM-THE-HARVARD-PROFESSOR-SIMON-GREENLEAF-WHICH-SUPPORT-THE-HISTORICAL-JESUS

As a side note, Chuck Colson was imprisoned for his involvement in Watergate prior to becoming a Christian. He said that the Watergate scandal was one of the things that contributed to his belief that the disciples' testimony about Jesus was true. The Watergate conspirators collaborated to conceal incriminating evidence. But once the truth began to leak out, each man scrambled to save himself. Jesus' disciples suffered persecution and torture for their testimony about him. People are unwilling to suffer to defend something they know to be false.

Normally, after the Romans crucified someone, the body was thrown into the city dump. In Jerusalem that place was called Gehenna. Sometimes it was used as an example of hell because it was continuously smoking from the fires and burning that never went out as more garbage was added to the piles. Interestingly, Jesus' body was not thrown into Gehenna. A rich man, Joseph of Arimathea, a follower of Jesus, asked the officials if he could have the body and Jesus was buried in the tomb Joseph intended for himself. This fulfilled the verse in Isaiah that predicted these exact events; "He had done no wrong and had never deceived anyone. But he was buried like a criminal; he was put in a rich man's grave."[83]

But Jesus did not stay dead. That's because he was innocent. Only sinners deserve death, "For the wages of sin is death, but the free gift of God is eternal life through Christ Jesus our Lord."[84] Because Jesus was innocent, he was able to die in the place of sinners, but because he was innocent and did not deserve the penalty of death himself, he did not stay dead, God raised him back to life.

That sounds incredible, and unbelievable. We don't see people who were clearly dead coming back to life. The first people who reported to Jesus' disciples that he was

[83] ISAIAH 53:9 (NLT)
[84] ROMANS 6:23 (NLT)

alive were not believed. But then, "He was seen by Peter and then by the Twelve (disciples). After that, he was seen by more than 500 of his followers at one time, most of whom are still alive, though some have died."[85] This is one of the reasons why people who examine the truth claims of the Bible, as one might examine a legal case, often come to the conclusion that the facts of the case prove that it is true. If two or three people claim to have witnessed the same event, and say the same thing about it, we assume they must be telling the truth. How about 500 witnesses?

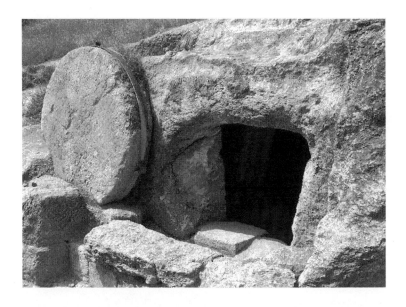

The empty tomb of Jesus

Jesus had 12 disciples who were with him continuously for 3 years and they were all witnesses to everything he said and did. All but one* of them died a violent death

---

[85] 1 CORINTHIANS 15:5-6 (NLT)
* THE APOSTLE JOHN DIED IN EXILE ON THE ISLAND OF PATMOS

because they would not deny what they saw and heard. They knew that their testimony was true and that Jesus was who he claimed to be. They would not deny it, even when threatened with an agonizing death. All they had to do to avoid torture and death would be to say they had made it all up, but none of them would do that. The Apostle Peter said, "For we were not making up clever stories when we told you about the powerful coming of our Lord Jesus Christ. We saw his majestic splendor with our own eyes."[86] There is much strong evidence that Christianity is true. The only reason people believe that there is not, is because the evidence has never been presented to them!

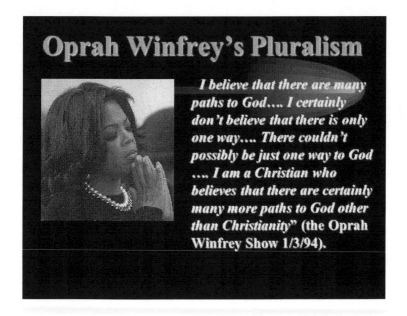

Oprah Winfrey says she's a Christian but she also believes Christianity is not the only path to God. Jesus would

---

[86] 2 PETER 1:16 (NLT)

strongly disagree with her. It would be nice to believe that all religions lead to God, but if you've ever compared the beliefs of world religions with Christianity, you recognize that is impossible, because they directly contradict each other in so many ways. Jesus said, "I am the way, the truth, and the life. No one can come to the Father except through me."[87] The thing to note here is that he did not say, "I am A way, A truth, A life" He claims to be *THE* way, the only way. "…for there is *one* God and *one* mediator between God and mankind, the man Christ Jesus, who gave himself as a ransom for all people."[88]

A popular belief today is that 'truth is relative.' I can believe one way and that's true for me, you can hold an opposite belief and that's true for you. Jesus claimed to be the *THE* truth, in fact just before his crucifixion he told Pontius Pilate that "I was born and came into the world to testify to the truth. All who love the truth recognize that what I say is true."[89] He also claimed to be the only path to God. Everyone is entitled to their opinion, but according to the Bible truth is not open to private preference. I might like to believe that gravity doesn't exist, and that 'my truth' is I can jump off a building and not get killed. But reality does not conform to me. I must conform to reality.

People really know that is true, and that's the way they live. "People live as if there is meaning, value, purpose and hope, even if their worldview provides no basis for that."[90] Cut in front of a long line at the grocery store and you will hear a unanimous, "That's not fair!" from the

---

[87] JOHN 14:6 (NLT)
[88] 1 TIMOTHY 2:5-6 (NLT)
[89] JOHN 18:37 (NLT)
[90] REFLECTIONS NEWSLETTER JUNE 2019

people behind you. Why not? Says who? If truth is relative they have no basis for objecting. They don't drive as if they can make up or change the rules of driving to what is 'true for them.' They know they have to conform to what the rules actually are or they'll get killed running a red light. So it's odd that they think they can arbitrarily invent a religion or assign attributes to God just because they want it to be true, as Oprah does. He is as He has described Himself to be in the Bible, not how we want Him to be.

Jesus claimed to be the only way, which excludes all other options. This is how C.S. Lewis described it in my favorite book, Mere Christianity;

"I am trying here to prevent anyone saying the really foolish thing that people often say about Him: I'm ready to accept Jesus as a great moral teacher, but I don't accept his claim to be God. That is the one thing we must not say. A man who was merely a man and said the sort of things Jesus said would not be a great moral teacher. He would either be a lunatic—on the level with the man who says he is a poached egg—or else he would be the Devil of Hell. You must make your choice. Either this man was, and is, the Son of God, or else a madman or something worse. You can shut him up for a fool, you can spit at him and kill him as a demon or you can fall at his feet and call him Lord and God, but let us not come with any patronizing nonsense about his being a great human teacher. He has not left that open to us. He did not intend to. . . . Now it seems to me obvious that He was neither a lunatic nor a fiend: and consequently, however strange or terrifying or unlikely it may seem, I have to accept the view that He was and is God". [91]

Lewis also wrote, "We may note in passing that He was never regarded as a mere moral teacher. He did not produce that effect on any of the people who actually met him. He produced mainly three effects — Hatred —Terror – Adoration. There was no trace of people expressing mild approval."[92]

THE GOSPEL

(GOD'S RESCUE OPERATION)

J.R.R. Tolkein, author of The Lord of the Rings, coined the term, eucatastrophe by affixing the Greek prefix eu, meaning good, to catastrophe (a good catastrophe). It is a sudden turn of events at the end of a story which ensures that the protagonist does not meet some terrible, impending, and very plausible and probable doom.[93] Jesus's entrance into time and space was a eucatastrophe; God dramatically rescuing humanity from impending doom.

"For God so loved the world, that He gave his only Son, that whoever believes in him should not perish but have

---

[91] MERE CHRISTIANITY BY C.S. LEWIS
[92] 1950 ESSAY, "WHAT ARE WE TO MAKE OF JESUS?" C.S. LEWIS
[93] HTTPS://EN.WIKIPEDIA.ORG/WIKI/EUCATASTROPHE

eternal life."[94] The last words Jesus spoke from the cross were, "It is finished!"[95] The actual word is tetelestai, which is an accounting term that means "paid in full." When Jesus uttered those words, He was declaring the debt we owed to His Father was wiped away completely and forever. Jesus eliminated the debt owed by mankind— the debt of sin. And so God could be just, and also justify (vindicate) those who have faith in Jesus [and rely confidently on Him as Savior]. [96] The word Gospel means 'Good News' and this is Good News indeed!

The Roman form of capital punishment in Jesus' day was crucifixion, a slow and excruciation form of death. He was placed on a cross between two convicted felons. One of them began to taunt Jesus and dared him to come off the cross and save himself. The other responded, "Don't you fear God even when you have been sentenced to die? We deserve to die for our crimes, but this man hasn't done anything wrong." Then he said, "Jesus, remember me when you come into your Kingdom." And Jesus replied, "I assure you, today you will be with me in paradise."[97]

To quote Phillip Yancy, "Jesus forgave a thief dangling on a cross, knowing full well the thief had converted out of plain fear. That thief would never study the Bible, never attend synagogue or church, and never make amends to those he had wronged. He simply said 'Jesus, remember me' And Jesus promised, 'Today you will be with me in paradise.' *It was another shocking reminder that grace does not depend on what we have done for God, but*

---

[94] JOHN 3:16 (NLT)
[95] JOHN 19:30 (NLT)

[96] ROMANS 3:26 (AMP)

[97] LUKE 23:40-43 (NLT)

rather on what God has done for us. "[98] All we need to do is accept it.

It took me a very long time to understand what the word 'grace' means in a Christian context. The more common, conversational definition of 'grace' is, "simple elegance or refinement of movement", so I didn't understand how that related to salvation. When Christians speak of 'God's grace' it's an entirely different use of the word. It comes from the Greek word, caris. The basic idea is simply, "non-meritorious or unearned favor, an unearned gift, a favor or blessings bestowed as a gift, freely and *NEVER as merit for work performed.*"

Theological grace is *"that which God does for mankind through His Son, which mankind cannot earn, does not deserve, and will never merit."*

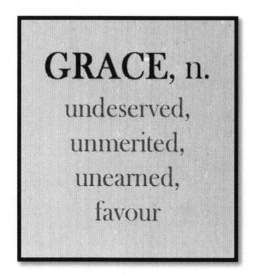

Grace is a word that rubs us the wrong way. It's a continual struggle to remember and believe it to be true, because we think much more highly of ourselves than we

---

[98] HTTPS://ME.ME/I/JESUS-FORGAVE-A-THIEF-DANGLING-ON-A-CROSS-KNOWING-FULL-7590097

ought to think. We think we are better, stronger, nobler and more capable than we really are. We want to be in control and 'pull ourselves up by our own bootstraps.' We have been taught from the time we were infants that if we are good we earn rewards and if we are bad we earn punishment and it's very hard to break that line of thought.

We are not basically good, God does not grade on the curve. His standard is perfection, and we are powerless to get back on his good side by doing good works, no matter how many good things we do. And so God did all the work and we bring nothing to the table, nothing! "For it is by grace you have been saved, through faith—and this is not from yourselves, it is the gift of God—not by works, so that no one can boast."[99] *Salvation is a gift of God's grace, plus nothing. We just have to accept it by faith and it's ours.*

At this point you might be thinking, "Wait a minute! That's crazy! Aren't Christians supposed to do good works, like feeding the poor, watching out for widows and orphans, taking care of the sick and many other good works?" That is absolutely correct; Christians are supposed to love others and do good works. The Bible says, "What good is it, dear brothers and sisters, if you say you have faith but don't show it by your actions? Can that kind of faith save anyone?"[100] "Faith by itself, if it is not accompanied by action, is dead." [101] The Protestant Reformer, Martin Luther, strongly affirmed that "It is faith alone that saves, but faith that saves is never alone."[102] The reason that faith without works is of no value is only because faith without corresponding works isn't faith at all!

---

[99] EPHESIANS 2:8-9 (NLT)
[100] JAMES 2:14 (NLT)
[101] JAMES 2:17 (NIV)
[102] HTTPS://WWW.GOODREADS.COM/QUOTES/26222-WE-ARE-SAVED-BY-FAITH-ALONE-BUT-THE-FAITH-THAT

If I were in a crowded theater and the smell of smoke filled the air followed by an announcement that the building was on fire, if I believed (had faith) that was a true statement I would quickly get up and get out of the building as rapidly as possible. I would take immediate action. That would demonstrate that I actually believed the building was on fire.

On the other hand, if I smelled the smoke and heard the announcement and then just sat there quietly waiting for the movie to start, then I would either be insane or it would be clear that I didn't believe the announcement and I thought the whole thing was a hoax. We demonstrate our beliefs by our actions.

> If we really believe something, we will act according to that belief.

"How can you show me your faith if you don't have good deeds? I will show you my faith by my good deeds."[103] If we claim to believe we are sinners and that God saved us, then we owe Him everything! But we have nothing to offer in return, we can't possibly pay Him back. Our good works buy us nothing at all. In fact it's insulting to say that God paid such a high price for our salvation by sending His son to take our punishment and in exchange gave us his righteousness and now we have to add something to that. By saying we must add our good works we are also

---

[103] JAMES 2:18 (NLT)

saying that Christ's sacrifice was not good enough. That's one reason the Bible says, "God resists the proud but gives grace to the humble."[104] Pride is a feeling of deep pleasure or satisfaction derived from one's own achievements. If we want to rely on our own achievements and good works instead of God's mercy and grace, He will resist us.

"Jesus told this story to some who had great confidence in their own righteousness and scorned everyone else: 'Two men went to the Temple to pray. One was a Pharisee, and the other was a despised tax collector. The Pharisee stood by himself and prayed this prayer: 'I thank you, God, that I am not like other people—cheaters, sinners, adulterers. I'm certainly not like that tax collector! I fast twice a week, and I give you a tenth of my income.'

"But the tax collector stood at a distance and dared not even lift his eyes to heaven as he prayed. Instead, he beat his chest in sorrow, saying, 'O God, be merciful to me, for I am a sinner.' I tell you, this sinner, not the Pharisee, returned home justified before God. For those who exalt themselves will be humbled, and those who humble themselves will be exalted." [105]

If there was any other way to redeem mankind, Jesus asked in prayer to use that other way. "He went on a little farther and bowed with his face to the ground, praying, "My Father! If it is possible, let this cup of suffering be taken away from me. Yet I want your will to be done, not mine." [106] The events following His prayer show that there was no other way; Jesus Christ is the only possible

---

[104] JAMES 4:6 (NLT)

[105] LUKE 18:9-18 (NLT)
[106] MATTHEW 26:39 (NLT)

sacrifice to make us right with God. "If keeping the law could make us right with God, then there was no need for Christ to die."[107] Humankind originally had only one law to keep, but they could not or would not. We are law breakers, not law keepers. Tell me I cannot walk on the grass or "do not touch, wet paint," and those are exactly the things I have an impulse to do. We are not saved by our works, but by our faith in His work for us. But we should notice a change in people who call themselves Christians. The works prove that we truly believe what God has done for us.

Larry Flynt illustrates this point. He published the pornographic magazine, "Hustler" and was a self-proclaimed atheist until 1977 when Larry claimed to have become an evangelical Christian, saying he was 'born again.' However nothing changed, he continued to publish his pornographic magazine, and kept his strip clubs open. If he truly believed the words of Jesus and had truly been 'born again' as he claimed, there would have been corresponding actions, or works, to support that claim.

Larry might not change overnight, but he would have been uncomfortable with the business he was in and sought to get out of it. But getting out of the porn business would not have saved him; it would only have revealed that he had a true change of heart and that he had faith. So it comes as no surprise that today he once again considers himself to be an atheist, not because he didn't have works, but because he never had genuine faith to begin with.

By his sacrifice Jesus made peace between man and God, but it can only be appropriated if we accept it. Someone may give you a gift, but if you refuse to open it or accept it, then you don't have the gift, even though it was

---

[107] GALATIANS 2:21 (NLT)

intended for you and could have and would have been yours. If we reject God's provision, we are hopelessly lost because according to the Bible there is no other way. No plan B.

God has done so much at infinite cost to Himself to rescue us from judgment, and make peace between Himself and us. If we say, 'no thanks, I'm a good person, I don't need it, don't want it, I can take care of myself,' "What makes us think we can escape if we ignore this great salvation that was first announced by the Lord Jesus himself..."[108] "How much more severely do you think someone deserves to be punished who has trampled the Son of God underfoot, who has treated as an unholy thing the blood of the covenant that sanctified them, and who has insulted the Spirit of grace?"[109] In other words we must trample over Christ's body, God's gracious offer and everything he did to save us in order to end up in hell. God doesn't want us to go there, He did all the work to prevent it from happening, and if we say, 'no thanks,' all we have left is His justified anger.

Hell is an unpleasant subject, but many people are unconcerned about it because they have convinced themselves that it doesn't exist. It's interesting to note that Jesus spoke more about hell more than any other person in the Bible. In fact, Jesus talked about hell more than he talked about heaven and described hell in greater detail. He said it is a place of eternal torment (Luke 16:23), of unquenchable fire (Mark 9:43) where people will gnash their teeth in anguish and regret (Matthew 13:42), and from which there is no return, even to warn loved ones (Luke 15:19-31). He calls hell a place of "outer darkness" (Matthew 25:30). Jesus knew, believed, and warned about the reality of hell.

---

[108] HEBREWS 2:3 (NLT)
[109] HEBREWS 10:29 (NIV)

But hell was not made for human beings. Jesus said that the eternal fire of hell was "prepared for the devil and his angels" (Matthew 25:41). People were made for God. Hell was made for the Devil. Yet people who die in their sin, without Jesus Christ as Lord and Savior, will spend eternity in hell with the one Being (Satan) who is most unlike God.

We all know a handful of people we love and strongly desire to be with. But imagine if someone far more intelligent than Einstein, more regal than Queen Elizabeth, richer than Bill Gates, and much more powerful than any president, felt that way about you? God is all of those things and so much more, and surprisingly He loves us and went to great lengths to make it possible for us to have a relationship with Him! He wants you to be with Him. But do you want to be with Him? Ultimately, 'The gospel is not a way to get people to heaven; it is a way to get people to God.'[110] It's a way of overcoming every obstacle to everlasting friendship and joy with God. Wow!

Dr. Ken Boa frequently says, "In the end there are two types of people; those who seek after God, and those who seek to avoid Him. They will both succeed." C.S. Lewis said, "I willingly believe that the damned are, in one sense, successful rebels to the end; that the doors of hell are locked on the inside,"[111] and "There are only two kinds of people in the end: those who say to God, 'Thy will be done,' and those to whom God says, in the end, 'Thy will be done.' All that are in Hell, choose it. Without that self-choice there could be no Hell. No soul that seriously and

[110] HTTPS://WWW.GOODREADS.COM/WORK/QUOTES/26568 9-GOD-IS-THE-GOSPEL-MEDITATIONS-ON-GOD-S-LOVE-AS-THE-GIFT-OF-HIMSELF
[111] THE PROBLEM OF PAIN BY C.S. LEWIS

constantly desires joy will ever miss it. Those who seek find. To those who knock it is opened."[112]

We have all been extended God's gracious invitation of forgiveness and eternal life. It is freely available to all. If you would entrust your life into God's loving hands you can have peace with God and assurance of eternal life; all you have to do is ask Him. For "everyone who calls on the name of the Lord will be saved."[113] God is offering you a free gift and you just need to receive it. Then life's disasters will not overwhelm you, and whether you live or die you cannot lose. You are eternally secure and have peace with God, starting right now.

[112] THE GREAT DIVORCE BY C.S. LEWIS
[113] ROMANS 10:13 (NLT)

EPILOGUE

I can't tell you how many times I thought I had finished writing this book when I learned something new or thought of something else that should be included. I have only scratched the tip of the iceberg, there is so much more that could and should be said and I would urge you to continue to learn more.

If you have given your life to Christ, that is only the beginning. Again, quoting C.S. Lewis, "We have to be continually reminded of what we believe. Neither this belief nor any other will automatically remain alive in the mind. It must be fed. And as a matter of fact, if you examined a hundred people who had lost their faith in Christianity, I wonder how many of them would turn out to have been reasoned out of it by honest argument? Do not most people simply drift away?"[114]

And so it's very important to continue to learn and grow in your understanding. Christianity is a relationship with the Creator of the Universe. Like all living things, if faith is not fed and cared for, it dies away. So it is important to find a good church. Not just any church, but one that teaches the Bible. I've been to many different churches and I find that some churches teach the Bible much better than others.

You should also pray and read the Bible yourself. And don't just read to get points with God and get it over with as soon as possible. As with any other book, it is better to read a little with your mind engaged and thinking about

---

[114] p. 123, 124 MERE CHRISTIANITY

what you are reading than to read many pages without understanding.

There are many excellent translations of the Bible. One of the oldest and perhaps the best known is the King James Version (KJV). It is a very precise and even artistic translation of the Bible. The KJV was completed in 1611 during the lifetime of Shakespeare, so the language style can sometimes be a little more difficult to understand, like watching one of Shakespeare's plays. I've read the KJV several times and it's not that difficult when you get used to it, but it's not the way we talk today. Just as I had difficulty understanding Hamlet's soliloquy, you may have to work harder if you choose that translation, which might be discouraging.

Since the meaning of words sometimes change over time, the New King James Version (NKJV) was produced as an effort to preserve the precision of the KJV but replace outdated, obsolete words with words in use today that are the equivalent. For example, in Old English the word, 'conversation' did not mean a discussion, it meant 'manner of life'. So where the King James Bible uses the word 'conversation' the NKJV substitutes the words 'manner of life'. These word changes along with removing outdated words such as; thee, thou, ye, thine, doest, camest, goeth, etc. make it clearer for modern readers.

All the translations are basically saying the same things; the wording is just a little different. My favorite translation is the New Living Translation (NLT) because it reads like modern English; it is very simple and straightforward. Almost all of the Bible references used in this book were taken from the New Living Translation. If you would like to compare various translations try visiting biblegateway.com or biblehub.com. In fact, if you don't have a Bible you can read it on-line at those sites for free and 'try out' various translations until you find the one you like best.

When you start reading you could start at the beginning, Genesis. But if you have never read the Bible before, you might consider beginning with the Book of John in the New Testament. The Book of John contains many quotations of Jesus' actual words and teachings as well as basics about Christianity. John was one of Jesus' disciples (students) and his reason for compiling his book is, "...these are written so that you may continue to believe that Jesus is the Messiah, the Son of God, and that by believing in him you will have life by the power of his name." [115]

Besides the Bible, the book I personally have found most helpful in understanding basic Christianity is <u>Mere Christianity</u>, by C.S. Lewis, and I heartily recommend it. Originally it was a series of BBC radio talks made by C.S. Lewis between 1941 and 1944, during the Second World War. It was the most popular radio program on the air with the exception of Winston Churchill's wartime speeches. The talks were adapted into the book and I've probably read it ten times or more. Once, before audio books were commonplace I even read and recorded it on cassette tape for Morris to listen to as a commuter. So that gives you some idea of how valuable I think it is. But while other books can be helpful, it is much more valuable to read the Bible itself, rather than books about the Bible.

---

[115] JOHN 20:31 (NLT)

Soli Deo Gloria

Surviving Cancer, Surprised by Life!

Printed in the United States of America

First Printing, 2019

ISBN 9781072979364

canylander@aol.com

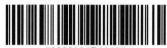

Made in the USA
Middletown, DE
06 August 2019